# COPING SUCCESSFULLY
## WITH PANIC ATTACKS

SHIRLEY TRICKETT trained as a nurse before becoming a counsellor and teacher. She has worked with anxious and depressed people for several years, and is the author of the successful *Coping with Anxiety and Depression* (Sheldon 1989). Her other books include *Irritable Bowel Syndrome and Diverticulosis* (Thorsons 1990; revd edn 1999) and *Coping with Candida* (Sheldon 1994). In 1987 she won a Whitbread Community Care Award.

# Overcoming Common Problems Series

*Selected titles*

A full list of titles is available from Sheldon Press,
36 Causton Street, London SW1P 4ST and on our website at
www.sheldonpress.co.uk

**Body Language: What you need to know**
David Cohen

**The Chronic Pain Diet Book**
Neville Shone

**The Complete Carer's Guide**
Bridget McCall

**The Confidence Book**
Gordon Lamont

**Coping Successfully with Psoriasis**
Christine Craggs-Hinton

**Coping Successfully with Varicose Veins**
Christine Craggs-Hinton

**Coping with Birth Trauma and Postnatal Depression**
Lucy Jolin

**Coping with Diabetes in Childhood and Adolescence**
Dr Philippa Kaye

**Coping with Family Stress**
Dr Peter Cheevers

**Coping with Hay Fever**
Christine Craggs-Hinton

**Coping with Kidney Disease**
Dr Tom Smith

**Coping with Polycystic Ovary Syndrome**
Christine Craggs-Hinton

**Coping with Tinnitus**
Christine Craggs-Hinton

**Coping with Your Partner's Death: Your bereavement guide**
Geoff Billings

**Every Woman's Guide to Digestive Health**
Jill Eckersley

**The Fertility Handbook**
Dr Philippa Kaye

**The Fibromyalgia Healing Diet**
Christine Craggs-Hinton

**Free Yourself from Depression**
Colin and Margaret Sutherland

**Helping Children Cope with Grief**
Rosemary Wells

**How to Be a Healthy Weight**
Philippa Pigache

**How to Get the Best from Your Doctor**
Dr Tom Smith

**The IBS Healing Plan**
Theresa Cheung

**Living with Birthmarks and Blemishes**
Gordon Lamont

**Living with Eczema**
Jill Eckersley

**Living with Schizophrenia**
Dr Neel Burton and Dr Phil Davison

**Living with a Seriously Ill Child**
Dr Jan Aldridge

**Osteoporosis: Prevent and treat**
Dr Tom Smith

**Overcoming Agoraphobia**
Melissa Murphy

**Overcoming Anorexia**
Professor J. Hubert Lacey, Christine Craggs-Hinton and Kate Robinson

**Overcoming Hurt**
Dr Windy Dryden

**Overcoming Insomnia**
Susan Elliot-Wright

**Overcoming Shyness and Social Anxiety**
Ruth Searle

**Overcoming Tiredness and Exhaustion**
Fiona Marshall

**Reducing Your Risk of Cancer**
Dr Terry Priestman

**Safe Dieting for Teens**
Linda Ojeda

**Stammering: Advice for all ages**
Renée Byrne and Louise Wright

**Stress-related Illness**
Dr Tim Cantopher

**Tranquillizers and Antidepressants: When to take them, how to stop**
Professor Malcolm Lader

**The Traveller's Good Health Guide**
Dr Ted Lankester

**Treating Arthritis – More Drug-Free Ways**
Margaret Hills

**Overcoming Common Problems**

# COPING SUCCESSFULLY
# WITH PANIC ATTACKS

## Shirley Trickett

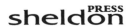

First published in Great Britain in 1992

Sheldon Press
36 Causton Street
London SW1P 4ST

Reprinted 8 times
Reissued 2009

The author and publisher have made every effort to ensure that
the external website addresses included in this book
are correct and up to date at the time of going to press. The author
and publisher are not responsible for the content, quality
or continuing accessibility of the sites.

Illustrations: Alasdair Smith (pages 67, 69, 87),
Tuffy Davies (page 31).

*British Library Cataloguing-in-Publication Data*
A catalogue record for this book is available from the British Library

ISBN 978–1–84709–071–3

1 3 5 7 9 10 8 6 4 2

Typeset by Deltatype Limited, Birkenhead, Merseyside
Printed in Great Britain by Ashford Colour Press

Produced on paper from sustainable forests

# Contents

# Important Note

This book is *not* a substitute for professional help. *Before* using self-help methods, you are strongly advised to take your health problems to your doctor. DIY diagnosis is foolish, and can be dangerous.

# Introduction

I trust you will find this an optimistic book with a commonsense approach to the very distressing problem of panic attacks. I have written it because I get so many requests for information on this subject. In it I seek to comfort, to reassure and to stress what I firmly believe, that panic attacks are *curable*. Yes, curable. I don't pretend that by reading the following chapters you are going to have all the answers, nor that the methods I describe are going to work overnight. What I do hope is that when you fully understand what is happening to you during a panic attack you will become less afraid and accept that they do not drop from the sky on to helpless people; there are always reasons for them.

## *You are causing your panic attacks*

I run the risk of you wanting to light the barbecue with this book before you read any further; *who* would want to give themselves these attacks? The full horror of a panic attack cannot be understood unless you have experienced one, so for me to suggest that you are responsible for the dreaded episodes could be irritating to say the least. I hope you will forgive this statement when I explain that I include myself in this. I rarely write about anything unless I have first-hand knowledge and I can assure you that I can describe a panic attack, in every fearful detail, from my own experience.

## *The experience of others*

I have also worked for ten years with people suffering from panic attacks and it is on this experience I draw to help you track down where your panic attacks are coming from. I trust you will also learn what you are doing to your body that is causing you to flush periodically with levels of adrenaline so abnormally high that your whole being reacts with fearsome and bizarre feelings. Such feelings quite understandably lead the sufferer to believe that the only possible outcome of the attack could be at least a heart attack, or stroke, and at worst sudden departure from this world. Here are some typical experiences of panic attacks.

John was away on a business course when he had his first (or what he thought of then as his first) panic attack. He was not worried about the course and was pleased he had been chosen. He was lying on his bed reading the paper when he began to feel breathless, sweaty and very frightened. He moved around and made a cup of coffee and it went away. The incident was repeated when he had to make an overnight stay to collect a visa. His mother had been a nervous person with agoraphobia so he recognized what he was feeling as nervous symptoms but was puzzled as to why they were happening. He loved his holidays and he enjoyed going out so he knew he was not agoraphobic.

It was not until he made the connection that it was only when he was alone and away from home (his holidays were spent with a girlfriend) that he began to understand. He recalled he had the same feelings as a child when he was sent to an aunt to recover from measles. He remembered feeling alone and afraid without his elder brother. The insight and talking about his early experience stopped the feelings.

Mary was a cheerful, capable woman of forty-nine. She was prescribed a sleeping pill when she was having difficulty sleeping after being made redundant. It was the first time she had taken pills for anything; in fact, her first visit to the doctor for many years. After a few days on the pills she began to feel 'jumpy' and depressed. After two weeks she had a panic attack while she was out shopping and two more followed the next day.

Her daughter said she had not been the same person since she took the sleeping pills and put them down the lavatory. Mary was annoyed at the time but thanked her a few days later. She had two sleepless nights, but the day after she stopped the pills she began to feel more like herself and had no further panic attacks.

Please note: Mary was able to stop her pills abruptly because she had only been on them two weeks. This cannot normally be done. More about this on pages 54–5.

Debbie was nineteen and worked in an office. She gave up drinking tea at work because she could not hold a cup without shaking. She also had difficulty swallowing and felt something awful was going to happen. This only happened at work. She was unhappy there because of a supervisor whom she considered to be unjust. She was frustrated because she was afraid to confront the woman.

She talked to a counsellor at her church and was able to see it was a repeat of a very painful earlier situation; another experience where she felt helpless. She had been brought up by her father and from when she was thirteen to sixteen years old his girlfriend had lived with them. The woman was unkind and domineering but Debbie's father did not seem to notice the situation. Debbie felt alone and frustrated.

After self-assertion classes she was able to confront her supervisor and as she slowly became more confident and in charge the feelings disappeared.

## Sharing the experience

It is often very difficult to convince someone that these symptoms are panic attacks, and even harder to get them to accept that they can take control and learn to manage them or get rid of them altogether. I find working with groups of people who suffer panic attacks very rewarding and effective. I could often talk myself hoarse in a one-to-one session without a great deal of success, only to find that when sufferers attend a group and listen to the experiences of a number of others they are instantly reassured. Some of these experiences are shared with you in this book. Several types of panic attacks are described in the hope that you will find one similar to your experience; but, remember, you are unlikely to find a mirror image of your own.

## *What this book has to offer*

The approach here is that of the physical management of anxiety: that is, how to regulate the breathing, the blood sugar levels, and how to release muscle spasm in order to slow down the production of adrenaline, the overproduction of which is the main cause of panic attacks. What happens to the body when the emergency button is being pressed continuously is discussed fully in Part One and self-help methods which will enable you to take your finger off the button are explained in Part Two. The suggestions in Part Two will not make sense unless you have understood why your body is behaving the way it is, so do not be tempted to turn straight to the self-help section. Part One will also help you to turn sleuth and track down where your symptoms are coming from. You could be surprised by some of the causes.

You don't have to be 'highly strung' to get panic attacks. Many people believe panic attacks are only experienced by people who are already over-anxious. This has not been my experience; I have seen many people who have suffered panic attacks which come from purely physical causes, for example dieting, prolonged exercise or reaction to a drug.

## *Working through the book*

Whilst the initial approach is through the body, emotional and spiritual health are also discussed. Wholeness comes from the harmony of body, mind and spirit but in saying that you have to start somewhere, and looking after the body paves the way to peace of mind which in turn allows you to connect with what I believe is the most important part of you: your soul, spirit, essence or inner being, whatever name it is given. The importance of unconditionally loving the person you find on your inner journey is the most important step towards wholeness.

The book also gives several medical references on the subject of hyperventilation, the main cause of panic attacks, and discusses why the symptoms are often dismissed or overlooked. If you are receiving medical treatment this book is not meant to replace it, but rather to work alongside it. What you might find,

4

however, is that when you are educated about your body and its responses you are able to reduce, or to come off, tranquillizers or antidepressants.

**Please note**: Do not make any changes in your medication without the approval of your doctor and without full instruction on withdrawal methods (see pages 54–7). It is also important not to use any of the dietary advice if it conflicts with a diet provided by your doctor.

# PART ONE
# Knowing Yourself

# 1
# The Dreaded Panic Attack

Men are flesh and blood and apprehensive.
Shakespeare, *Julius Caesar*

## *What is a panic attack?*

A panic attack is an exaggeration of the body's normal response to fear. The chemical adrenaline which is normally produced when we need action – to run from danger, to fight, or even to get angry – is overproduced, and the result is a multitude of unpleasant sensations and a distressing degree of fear. It is a pity that these feelings, because that is *all* they are, have been labelled panic attacks. The word attack suggests illness, something that has to be endured, an episode that the sufferer is powerless to avoid or control. It will be seen from the following chapters that this is not so. A better term would be 'adrenaline flushes' or 'adrenaline surges'. This describes exactly what is happening and sounds much less alarming.

### *What does it feel like to be overflowing with adrenaline?*

The body behaves like an old Charlie Chaplin film or a video on fast forward: everything is running at top speed, the breathing increases, the heartbeat gets faster, the blood pressure rises, and thoughts race around. Every system in the body is affected, including the digestion; hence one of greatest worries of the panic attack sufferer – the urgent need for the lavatory.

## *What does a panic attack feel like?*

Sandra:  I feel convinced something terrible is about to happen and I shake from head to foot. My mouth goes dry and I feel I can't swallow. It usually happens in a shop. When I get into the fresh air it goes off.

Mark:  I feel very weak as if I'm going to faint and I have trouble getting a good breath. I sweat and my girlfriend

9

says I go pale. I feel so helpless when it happens and I'm always convinced I'm dying. I feel such a fool afterwards.

Peter:      I feel suddenly overcome by terror, my heart races and I feel I want to run. I must get out of wherever I am and get home as quickly as possible; I never get them at home.

Marjory:    My thoughts are so weird and my words sound odd. I always feel as if I'm having a stroke. Everything around me looks strange. I seem to seize up with fear each time and it takes a lot to convince me at the time that it is just a panic attack. I'm willing to accept this later but not at the time, in fact I get quite irritated if anyone suggests that it is nerves.

Liam:       It's as though a sudden deep depression jumps out of nowhere. I'm anxious too but seem to be more aware of the gloom. I feel utterly hopeless when this happens and often miserable for a couple of days afterwards. When I have recovered and analyse it I can usually see that anxiety starts it off, although that does not occur to me at the time. I live in dread of another attack for a few days.

## Symptoms of a panic attack

This list is meant to be encouraging not daunting. It should convince you that this simple opening of the adrenaline floodgates can cause all those funny feelings you are getting, and more:

* *Fear.* Of dying, the world coming to an end, going mad, having a heart attack, having a stroke, losing control, fainting, being incontinent, being sick, shouting, looking foolish, running, the unknown.
* *Bewilderment.* When they are in the middle of it even a regular sufferer can find it difficult to accept that what they are experiencing is a panic attack.
* *Disorientation.* How did I get here?
* *Feelings of unreality.* Even a familiar setting looks strange.

10

- *Heightened perception.* Things around seem too fast, too loud, too bright.
- *Feelings of gloom and doom.* Sudden overwhelming feelings of sadness or grief.
- *Irritability.* Inability to cope with small irritations.
- *Dizziness.* I'm going to fall over.
- *Sweating.* I'm sweating, I'm ill.
- *Palpitations.* My heart is going to burst; I'm having a heart attack.
- *Tight chest.* I can't get my breath.
- *Pain in the chest.* It's a heart attack.
- *Ringing in the ears.* My head feels funny; it's a stroke.
- *Tingling in the hands, feet or around the mouth.* I'm having a stroke.
- *My tongue won't work.* I'm having a stroke.
- *I can't think of words.* I'm having a stroke; I'm going senile.
- *Fainting.* When the body can't take any more adrenaline an artificial relaxation response is produced by the brief unconsciousness of fainting; the muscles relax, the breathing slows, etc. Perhaps a panic attack could be the body pushing for this 'going for a faint'.

Note: Pain in the chest must *always* be investigated by a doctor.

## Who has panic attacks?

You, me, the man next door, his little boy; maybe even the Pope. We all run on adrenaline, therefore we could all suffer a panic attack at some time in our lives.

### Do you have to be an anxious person to have panic attacks?

No. If you are normally over-anxious you are more likely to have a panic attack than the person who is very relaxed, but as you will see from the list of causes of panic attacks there are some physical triggers which have nothing to do with anxiety levels.

### Helpful panic attacks

When there is real danger, say from an earthquake or an assailant, a panic attack would be a normal response; the person would run away or fight. The extra adrenaline could be used productively.

*Unhelpful panic attacks*

Here there is no recognizable threat; the sufferer is responding with extreme fear to a normal event, for example having to stand in a queue in the supermarket or go to a party. The trigger that starts the panic may be physical or emotional (this will be discussed later). Once again adrenaline floods the body to such an extent that it produces very unpleasant physical feelings and also a level of fear so disabling that the sufferer cannot make sense of what is happening and, worst of all, does not know what to do. He/she has no way to use the extra energy; how can he/she turn the adrenaline tap off? The person might want to run screaming from the queue or the party in the same way they would run from the earthquake but their rational mind knows there is no real danger. It's all very confusing. Unfortunately, the helpless feeling invoked sows the seed for the next panic attack and so the vicious circle is started.

*Occasional panic attacks*

These are often in response to certain situations, such as flying or a visit to the dentist, or they can be less specific and happen when the sufferer is 'run down'. They disappear when life is back on an even keel. Panic attacks caused by some physical triggers come into this group. For example, if a blocked nose causes overbreathing and panic, when the breathing returns to normal the attacks will disappear.

*Panic during and after stressful times*

People understand when they have panic attacks during times of crisis but are puzzled if they do not appear until after the stressful event: 'Jack is really well now; I'm not worried at all. Why should I have panic attacks now?' When the adrenaline levels have been raised to give more energy in a prolonged crisis they do not drop the instant they are no longer needed. The extra energy often discharges itself in panic attacks.

*Frequent panic attacks in the nervous person*

The person who is always anxious is more likely to have panic attacks. Life can be very limited for people who have panic attacks superimposed on a background of continuous anxiety. They are often agoraphobic and have social phobias. People in this group need professional help. The situation is not as bleak as it sounds and some people do very well. 'I have always been an anxious person' does not necessarily mean that is your fate for life. Patient teaching and long-term reassurance are a vital part of treatment.

## What are the causes of panic attacks?

They could be said to be:

- *Emotional*: exhausted nerves causing anxiety and depression.
- *Physical/emotional*: for example, exhausted nerves, causing muscle spasm or hyperventilation (overbreathing).
- *Physical*: for example, dieting, tight clothes.
- *Spiritual*: despair, no vision beyond a painful reality, death phobia.

It is quite difficult to put the causes of panic attacks under different headings because the effects of physical, emotional and spiritual discomfort can be interwoven. However, here is an attempt. We have seen that too much adrenaline causes the symptoms, but what can prompt the overproduction of this chemical? The list is quite long. Needless to say, we will not discuss anything which would reasonably cause a panic attack, such as finding a cobra in your compost heap.

### Physical causes

*Unstable blood sugar levels, dieting, fasting.* Why variations in the level of glucose in the blood cause panic attacks is fully discussed on pages 41–52.

*Inner ear problems.* Inner ear problems cause dizziness. It can be very frightening when the world suddenly starts to spin, particularly if it happens outside. An attack of vertigo (type of dizziness associated with inner ear problems) can lead to agoraphobia.

*Low blood pressure.* The French pay a great deal of attention to low blood pressure. It seems to go largely unnoticed here. It can however by a potent trigger for panic attacks because it can deprive the brain of oxygen causing anxiety, dizziness and fainting. Increasing salt consumption and taking more exercise can be helpful.

*Reactions to drugs.* Allergic reactions and side effects of some drugs can cause increased anxiety and panic attacks. Strangely enough tranquillizers and antidepressants can often do this, particularly at the beginning of treatment.

*Drug withdrawal, alcohol withdrawal, stopping smoking.* When any drug which sedates is withdrawn, adrenaline levels rise and panic attacks can occur (see pages 54–62).

*Chest hugging, tight clothing, chest problems.* Any restriction in the chest can lead to hyperventilation. This is the chief cause of panic attacks.

*Digestive problems, particularly food allergies.* Abnormal amounts of gas in the digestive system can push up on the diaphragm, restrict breathing and cause pain in the chest, both of which can trigger panic attacks.

I have covered food allergies, chemical sensitivities and candida in my book *Irritable Bowel Syndrome and Diverticulosis*. There are also many books in bookshops and health food shops which give detailed exclusion diets that enable you to discover which foods are affecting you. This problem is a great deal commoner than one would expect and since a reaction can produce palpitations, sweating and dizziness it is not surprising that it can cause feelings of panic. An Alka-Seltzer, or a teaspoon each of bicarbonate of soda and potassium bicarbonate in water (preferably warm), can 'turn off' the reaction. If you suffer from food allergies or intolerances it is often a sign that you need to clean your colon and change your diet. You could also benefit from vitamins, minerals and products such as acidophilus, which keep the gut bacteria in a state of balance. Digestive enzymes are also helpful. You could seek advice in your local health food store or ring or write to New Nutrition (see Useful Addresses). Helping your mind to ignore triggers for panic attacks is in the self-help section of the book.

*Stuffy nose.* This can lead to overbreathing and panic.

*Jet lag.* Fatigue and disruption can lead to raised anxiety levels.

*Chronic pain.* People in pain often hyperventilate in an attempt to control their discomfort. Unfortunately this also causes panic.

*Injections containing adrenaline.* Panic attacks have been reported after local anaesthetics at the dentist. Some local anaesthetic injections contain adrenaline.

*Stimulant prescribed drugs.* Appetite suppressants, steroids (whether they are taken for medical purposes or to boost athletic performance).

*Stimulant street drugs.* Including LSD, cocaine, cannabis.

*Heat, exercise.* An overheated room can cause a panic attack as can unaccustomed or violent exercise. Again the adrenaline levels are raised.

### Emotional/physical causes

Exhausted nerves, reduced activity after stressful events, over-breathing, frozen emotional pain (neurosis). These are all covered in the next two chapters.

*Child abuse.* People who have been physically, emotionally or sexually abused as children frequently suffer panic attacks in adult life.

This chapter should dispel the commonly held belief that only anxious peoples suffer panic attacks; *anything*, physical or emotional, which dramatically increases adrenaline levels can cause a panic attack. It is only when you understand this that they can be demystified and knocked down to size. The main cause of panic attacks, exhausted nerves, follows in the next chapter.

15

# 2

## Going to the Doctor
## with Panic Attacks

The ideal treatment (although there isn't much of it around!) would be anxiety management, where you would receive counselling and full education about what is going on in your body, breathing retraining, dietary advice, how to cope with chronic muscle tension, and so on. In addition, if your symptoms were very severe, perhaps the short-term, carefully supervised use of a tranquillizer or antidepressant could be offered.

### Does medication help panic attacks?

Tranquillizers, antidepressants and a drug called Tegretol are used for panic attacks and some people find them helpful. Others find drugs no help at all and many people have suffered a great deal through becoming chemically dependent on drugs which should not have been used long term. It must be remembered that whilst these drugs can be useful for some people in the short term they can actually be the cause of panic attacks and agoraphobia for others. This is discussed on pages 54–8.

### Does counselling work?

In part, yes, but psychology alone is not enough; the patient needs to be educated about what he/she is doing with his/her body. The 'counselling only' approach is a tortuous route to the patient's fears. Until the barriers of hyperventilation and muscle tension are broken down, the truth about the patient's problems can be inaccessible to patient and therapist.

## Compartmentalizing medicine

In these days of one doctor for this and one doctor for that frequently important things about a patient's condition get overlooked. For example, once a GP has referred a patient to a psychiatrist it seems the GP thinks his/her responsibilities are over. Whilst on the other hand the psychiatrist, who might have before him/her a woman with glaring nutritional deficiencies – woefully thin, a muddy skin and dull hair, cracks at the corners of her mouth – does not notice these things because he/she sees anything other than her psychological problems as the province of the GP.

## Through the body to the mind

If only the body/mind approach were more widely acknowledged in psychiatry, if the whole person were considered, it could change the face of modern adult psychiatric medicine. I feel strongly that change is needed, after ten years of seeing patients for whom the present system has been such a miserable failure.

I feel the people particularly at risk in the system are those who have less severe (but still very distressing) symptoms of anxiety and depression (including panic attacks); people who function well enough to avoid hospital admission; people who have had years of their lives wiped out and anxiety problems increased by being prescribed tranquillizers. The system also fails countless people who have their anxiety levels doubled and their own worth demolished by a six-week wait for a ten-minute appointment with a psychiatrist who is so rushed that the consultation must be as unrewarding as it is unhelpful to the patient:

> I am in and out in a flash; he looks at my notes all the time, answers the phone and then just says keep on with the tablets. There is so much I want to ask but there is not enough time. I am shaking all over with anger and frustration when I come out. I usually go to the outpatient lavatory for a good cry. That seems to help. I keep on thinking why bother going, but since this is all there is I just keep the appointments. (Thirty-six-year-old lawyer)

> I am only in a few minutes; he asks me about the sleeping pills and then I go for relaxation therapy. I lie down in a room and then the nurse or cleaner puts a tape on. When it finishes they come back and then I go home. I don't feel this is doing much; should I continue? (Forty-nine-year-old unemployed steel worker)

He always gets my name wrong, asks if he can tape the consultation (this makes me tongue-tied but I say yes) and then he repeats the questions he asked at the last session. My sex life does not seem of great importance to me at the moment; I'm far more worried about feeling well enough to finish my degree. He does not seem to hear this. I wish he would listen. (Twenty-two-year-old male student)

I have seen both a psychiatrist and a psychologist and neither taught me what I really wanted to know – what was actually going on in my body to give me such bizarre feelings. I have always been healthy and have very little medical awareness. I was pretty scared. I did not need to be told I had anxiety symptoms: I was living with them. I wanted to know *why* my hands and feet buzzed and why I felt so spaced out. I thought it must be multiple sclerosis.

I would not have needed a psychiatrist if I had understood what overbreathing and not eating properly could do to my brain. I have wasted two years of my life through their blinkered psychological attitude. They could only focus on my early life and the row with my boyfriend. I'm quite sure in my own mind now that the pain from the slipped disc started the habit of overbreathing and everything stemmed from that. I feel relieved, but angry that I did not know this at the beginning. (Thirty-two-year-old art historian)

These are not exaggerated experiences; I could fill the book with them. It is interesting to note that doctors who make half-hour weekly counselling appointments for stressed patients often seem to achieve very much better results than those of the hospital outpatient psychiatric departments.

### How could the system be improved?

Only by making stress 'respectable'. Generally people feel they have to have something worthy of a diagnostic label before they go to the doctor; what is really needed is a readily accessible nurse-therapist in the doctor's surgery. Not the nurse who takes out stitches and gives injections, but one who is trained in stress management; one who can get to the shoulder of a tense person *before* it freezes and massage it with an essential oil; one whose knowledge of health education goes beyond 'stop smoking, take exercise and cut down on fat'; one who can teach deep relaxation methods; one who can reassure the patient that the treatment will continue until he/she feels confident (not 'This is a stress management course – it lasts six weeks') – then you will have a prescription ten times safer and ten times more effective than anxiolytic drugs.

I am not saying tranquillizers and sleeping pills do not have their place in the very short term – they do – but in the long term they do a great deal more harm than good. Not only are they highly addictive for many people, but they also cause a multitude of physical and emotional problems, including depression. They also deny the patient the opportunity to learn that he/she can take charge of his/her nervous system, can regain self regard and, most importantly, can break the cycle. Patients will not live in fear of another attack of 'nerves' because they know if they deal with the early signs of stress this is not going to happen again, or even if individuals are neglectful enough to let it happen, they will have the knowledge that they came through it on a previous occasion and can do it again.

I am not suggesting that conventional medicine is superfluous; I believe that medical science and complementary medicine can often work hand in hand. What I do believe is harmful is to fail to consider the whole organism, to put health into compartments: a pill for this bit of you; cut out this offending bit of you, and hey presto you are cured. Dealing with the symptoms seems to be the priority without thought to the cause of the dis-ease and disharmony of the whole person.

Medical progress has cost us a lot, including the near extinction of the medicine woman, the village grandmother or the old lady who lived in the wood. The one who would give you 'opening medicine', a bowl of broth, massage your aches and pains, and comfort you with wisdom that reflected her deep spirituality – that's holistic medicine. 'Love is the highest level of medicine' (Paracelsus).

## *Will helping myself work?*

Yes, definitely. But remember self-help programmes can be

19

tedious. You are going to have to be prepared to make changes in your life and some of them are boring and time consuming. You will get discouraged at times, particularly if your symptoms are coming from wayward nerves which can take time to retrain. It can also take time to restore the body to a balanced state after illness or strict dieting. Be patient.

# 3

# Exhausted Nerves and Panic Attacks

You could be forgiven for saying this writer drones on and on about exhausted, overstimulated or oversensitized nerves in all her books; you are quite correct, I do, because to abuse the nervous system is the easiest way to disrupt your whole life. With shame I admit I do not always practise what I preach on this one, although of late I am trying to reform.

If you are too hard on your nerves, the adrenaline levels rise and all the funny (and awful) things start to happen. You are not just getting overtired and making muscles ache, you are altering brain chemistry. Inevitable a change of mood and, eventually, personality ensues.

Imagine a picture of a violin: the strings are taut, the player is plucking the strings in a frenzied pizzicato; you are the player, and the tight strings are your nervous system – if you pick it, it will never get better! Sorry about the pun, but I thought this image just might make you see what you are doing to yourself. Would you jump repeatedly on a compound fracture of your lower leg?

## Are raised adrenaline levels always negative?

No. This is what pushes you to win the egg and spoon race; this is what gives you the extra energy to stay up late studying for your finals, or gives you enough pep to clean the house, weed the garden, do the ironing, *and* produce the perfect Victoria sponge for a visiting relative. When the levels of adrenaline don't fall naturally after the stressful event, and there is more stress, this is when the damage is done. You have to guard against the habit of tension. You can only do this by bringing what you are doing into your conscious mind. This is why people like me spend hours on computers, getting more tense by the second to give you this vital information.

## What happens to my body when I am punishing my nerves?

Most of the physical signs show that your flight or fight response is overworking. How to correct this is discussed later.

- *Sweating*. This is usually the hands or under the arms, but some people say they pour with sweat all over.
- *Palpitations*. A symptom which worries most people; my heart beats wildly and seems to skip beats.
- *Digestive upsets*. Wind, heartburn, bloating, constipation or diarrhoea.
- *Changes in appetite*. Either loss of interest in food or compulsive eating.
- *Urinary problems*. All bodily functions are speeded up, including urination. There can be urgency where there is very little warning or frequent need for the lavatory.
- *Blood sugar problems*. Overstimulated nerves include the nerves to the pancreas resulting in the overproduction of insulin. This is the opposite of, but can also be the forerunner of, diabetes. The result is increased anxiety often associated with hunger, panic, blurred vision, twitching in the eyelid muscles, lightheadedness, headaches, sugar craving, wanting food an hour after a heavy meal, waking in the night between two and three a.m., feelings of inner trembling but no visible shaking, cold hands and feet, sudden low mood. More about this on pages 41–52.
- *Skin problems*. The lymphatic system (the garbage disposal system which clears out some of the waste products of metabolism) needs normal muscular action to function properly. If you are still and tense, toxins are not eliminated successfully through the skin – result, spots.

### Chronic muscle spasm

- *Headaches*. Tension in the scalp is the cause of the common tight band headache. Neck and shoulder tension causes the dull ache around the base of the skull and a feeling of being vague or depressed.
- *Neck and shoulder tension*. The neck is the gateway to the

22

head. If the neck and shoulder muscles are tight, the circulation to the head is restricted. It's like putting a ligature around your neck. This can cause:
  • Dizziness
  • Ringing in the ears
  • Blurred vision
  • Sinus problems.
• *Back aches*. When the muscles at the sides of the neck are tense this alters the position of the head which transfers the tension all the way down the spine.
• *Wobbly legs*. The legs can't work properly if the spine is out of alignment.
• *Shaking*. The body is geared for action and this need has not been met. Shaking expends this energy.
• *Tight chest*. Usually the result of overbreathing (see next chapter).
• *Loss of interest in sex*. With every system in the body disrupted it would be surprising if the hormones were not affected. In addition, with so much energy going into tension, and the body trying to balance on a spine that is being pulled in all directions, there can't be enough energy left for sex. Fear also causes loss of libido.
• *Insomnia*. When you understand what is going on in your body you will see that insomnia is an inevitable physiological result of what you are doing to your body and mind during the day. It is not another mysterious condition over which you have no control.

## *Emotional signs of frayed nerves*

• *Irritability*. Being annoyed by things that would not normally bother you, the queue moving slowly, the packet of biscuits that refuses to open without scissors, a teasing remark (even from a loved one), a wrong number.
• *Confusion*. Have I given the cat his pill? Yes I have, no I haven't. Telephone numbers you have known for years are suddenly erased from your memory. You buy a newspaper; you had already bought one when you shopped earlier. You're embarrassed by forgetting people's names.

- *Restlessness*. If you're in you want to be out; if you're out you want to be in.
- *Hyperactivity*. Doing several things at once at top speed.
- *Rapid speech*. You can hear yourself going on and on but you can't seem to control it.
- *Rapid thoughts*. Mind like a grasshopper, jumping from one thing to the next. The same line of a song running through your head.
- *Paranoia*. Feeling people don't like you or are talking about you. You don't like yourself much at the moment, do you? Perhaps that's why you think others are avoiding you.
- *Phobias*. Being afraid of things which do not normally worry you, such as going shopping or staying in a strange place.
- *Feelings of gloom and doom*. Morbid thoughts; you know they are silly but they still come.
- *Crying easily*. Bursting into tears when you bang your elbow, at a sudden noise, or even at a sentence in a book. Your emotions surface easily.
- *Fainting*. Useful discharge of pent-up energy in fearful or emotionally charged situations.

## How have I got into this state?

You have ignored your basic needs either by pushing your body or mind too far or by not listening to your inner being, your soul, your spirit, whatever you will call your essence. Or perhaps you have done all of these things.

### Physically punishing yourself

Do you push yourself to work just that extra half hour and then the extra thirty minutes become an hour? Do you watch how you are sitting or standing and take frequent breaks from your working position and repetitive movements? Do you take quick fixes, coffee, tea, cigarettes, chocolate, alcohol or drugs instead of well spaced regular meals? Do you breathe enough to keep you clear headed and healthy or just enough to stop you fainting? Do you continually take on more than you can reasonably cope with? Are you incapable of seeing your own needs and saying 'no'? Do you deprive yourself of fresh air, light and exercise?

### Brain fatigue

Can you ever just 'be' and do nothing at all, or do you imagine you are resting if you merely sit in an easy chair away from your work place: 'I'll just look at this report'; 'I'll just write to ...'; 'I'll just mend ...'? Do you ever give your mind a small space, when it is not being pushed around by you, to repair, to drift? Are you afraid to stop?

### Soul starvation

Do you ignore the promptings of your higher self, your intuitive knowledge, the guidance of your dreams? Do you deny your spirituality? Do you confuse religion and spirituality and dismiss them both? There will be more about paying attention to your inner being later.

## Summing up

In this chapter some of the causes of panic attacks have been discussed and we have seen that the most common cause is exhausted nerves. Very much associated with this condition is overbreathing or hyperventilation. This is the subject of the next chapter.

# 4
## Half-Breathe – Half-Live

### *Panic attacks and overbreathing (hyperventilation)*

This is a happy chapter; it's not going to give you dreary statistics; it's not going to shout death to chocolate cake or port; it is merely going to explain how poor breathing habits can not only make you feel dizzy, tired and vaguely unwell, but also how they can cause severe symptoms (including panic attacks) which can mimic most known diseases. These symptoms are often the cause of much misdiagnosis. The effects of overbreathing can range from feeling a little dizzy or being 'spaced out', having a tight throat or bloated abdomen, to severe chest pain, panic attacks, feeling unreal, anxiety, depression and muscle and joint pains. Overbreathing or hyperventilation can also complicate the picture where there is known organic disease. Hyperventilation is an important subject; six to eleven per cent of all patients seen in general practice breathe in this unhealthy way.

### *Calming the breath to control hyperventilation*

I thought it would be less confusing to include this simple way of breathing here rather than with the breathing exercises described in Part Two. Learning this simple method is the first step to overcoming hyperventilation and panic.

The principle is very simple. All you have to do is to make your *out* breath longer than your *in* breath.

1. Breathe in quickly but gently (preferably through the nose) for a count of 2 or 3. Do not take deep, gulping breaths. Do not hold your breath. Then:
2. Breathe out gently (letting the jaw go slack) to a count of 4 or 6. Do not blow out hard or force it.

After a few weeks' practice you can make the out breath even longer and get a gentle rhythm going of: *in* 1, 2, 3 *out* 1, 2, 3, 4, 5, 6, 7, 8, 9. Take it easy; it will take time to get to this stage. You will soon start to feel in control using this simple method.

This simple yoga breath (*pranayama*) is recommended by the *Journal of Psychosomatic Research* 28, pp. 265–73, for the control of symptoms of hyperventilation.

## What is overbreathing?

This is breathing in excess of the body's requirements. It is characterized by rapid respirations from the upper chest with marked variations in the rhythm and rate, often with frequent sighing or the need to take an occasional deep breath. It is sometimes called shoulder or collar bone breathing. Because such a small amount of the lung capacity is being used the breathing pattern produces changes in carbon dioxide levels in the blood and this seriously disrupts the function of the nervous system. The resulting disturbance in brain chemistry alters perception and the sufferer is unable to make sense of what he/she sees and hears. The symptoms can be bizarre and are so frightening that they trigger further panic attacks. Even if the neurological effects caused by a fall in the carbon dioxide levels are not severe enough to cause panic attacks, the continuous stress on the nervous system can lead to nervous exhaustion.

## What causes overbreathing?

Pain, fear, anything which constricts the chest such as tight clothing or cramped posture, gas in the stomach or bowel, stuffy nose, pain, excitement or compulsive talking. Deficiency of the B vitamins and a poor nutritional state could be another factor. A high sugar diet can also be a cause. This will be explained later.

- *Anxiety.*
  It is natural for the breathing to speed up when we need action. When we are in an anxious state the breathing mechanism is always in a state half-way to red alert.
- *Constriction of the chest.*
  Anything which does not allow full expansion of the chest such as tight clothing, muscular tension, posture, working in a confined space, and broken ribs.
- *Breathing difficulties.*
  Some chest conditions such as pleurisy, or upper respiratory

problems which cause a blocked nose make the sufferer take small breaths through the mouth.

• *Chronic muscular tension.*
This is an important cause of the problem. Not only are the muscles of respiration, the diaphragm and chest muscles, involved but the sternomastoid muscles are also implicated. One end of these runs from behind the ear to the upper end of the breastbone and the other end runs from the collar bone to the base of the skull. These muscles help to lift the collar bones and breastbone. They are an important part of the breathing mechanism and we will see later in the work part of the book why it is so important to avoid tension in these muscles. If they cannot rest at their full length, in addition to affecting the breathing, they can cause ear, sinus, throat and allergy problems.

## Can hyperventilation be corrected?

Yes. The symptoms disappear when normal breathing patterns are established. More about this later.

When you read the list of symptoms caused by hyperventilation you will see that many of them are identical to the feelings of a panic attack. I can hear you saying: 'I can understand a soldier in combat being so afraid that he overbreathes enough to have a panic attack [see page 38] but I should not be afraid in the supermarket. Why does it happen to me? How can I be hyperventilating?' The answer is that if the fear is coming from your subconscious you may not be able to make sense of it, but if it happens repeatedly in the same situation you may have to accept that something is triggering your fear and this causes you to overbreathe and then to panic.

It is interesting to note that recent research has found that even when a diagnosis of 'neurocirculatory asthenia' has been reached, the role of hyperventilation may nevertheless go unnoticed. It follows therefore that neither will the correct treatment (breathing retraining) be given (see 'Hyperventilation Syndromes: Infrequently recognised expressions of anxiety and stress', by Gregory J. Magrian, *Medicine* 61, no. 4).

## Do people know about overbreathing?

As a result of articles in the popular press public awareness is growing, but unfortunately medical awareness is still in its infancy. Few doctors notice the subtle but extremely common symptom picture of the low-grade habitual hyperventilator and are only aware of the severe symptoms (difficulty breathing and tetany, a claw-like muscle spasm of the hands) of overt hyperventilation. Why is this so? Is it because the subject is given little importance in the medical curricula? Is it because the symptoms mimic so many conditions and medical practitioners are always looking for organic disease? Or is it that the ever-handy diagnosis of anxiety or depression conveniently solves the problem and the tranquillizers or antidepressants often prescribed coincidentally relieve some of the symptoms?

Could it be that some doctors feel this subject to be 'old hat' and skip over the coverage in medical journals, or has perhaps documentation on the subject been around too long? Whatever the reason, judging by the numbers of people who undergo unnecessary neurological, cardiac and respiratory investigations, it is a condition that is repeatedly overlooked. This is a great pity because a simple test – the provocation test – in which the patient is asked to overbreathe for two to three minutes, can confirm the diagnosis of hyperventilation. The symptoms are then compared with those the sufferer experiences during a panic attack. This simple test would save a lot of anxiety and a lot of NHS money. Doctors are often as baffled as the patient by the strange symptoms but do not consider hyperventilation as a cause. An article in the *Journal of the Royal Society of Medicine* suggests that we have seen a remarkable upsurge of interest in the role of hyperventilation in anxiety, panic and phobic states. There may have been more academic interest but little practical help is available. It is rare for a patient to be taught breathing retraining in General Practice. It could be done, and it would cut down the need for prescriptions for tranquillizers and antidepressants.

## Is it difficult to spot the chronic hyperventilator?

To be fair, the chronic hyperventilator does often have the

symptoms of anxiety and depression but this still cannot excuse the frequency with which the clear physical manifestations of hyperventilation are missed.

## Chicken or egg?

Which comes first? Does the hyperventilation cause the anxiety symptoms or does the anxiety cause symptoms of the hyperventilation? It would appear by the dearth of treatment for overbreathing that most practitioners accept the latter, although Professor L. C. Lum, an expert on this subject, did much to promote the role of hyperventilation in anxiety disorders, often dismissed by the medical profession.

## Educating the sufferer

The first step in helping someone who hyperventilates is to convince them that their symptoms are coming from shallow breathing. This is often not an easy task. Some sufferers dismiss the suggestion as being too simple an answer, others become wary and feel an element of blame. The sufferer needs to be reassured that breathing in excess of the body's requirements produces a far from simple chain of physiological events which are so complex that many systems in the body can be disrupted. If the sufferer argues that they don't normally breathe at the rate of the provocation test it should be explained that even two breaths per minute more than the body needs can produce symptoms.

When people feel they are being accused of hysterical hyperventilation it is useful to explain that it would be hard to do that during sleep, which many people do. This is why it is possible to wake up with a panic attack.

Once the sufferer is convinced overbreathing is causing the symptoms (this may take more than one provocation test), the person is taught to respond to stress with slow breathing – breathing retraining (more about this later). This is not an overnight cure; it often takes weeks of tedious effort.

To tell the patient there is nothing wrong is not reassuring, it causes more anxiety. It suggests to people either that they have some serious complaint that defies diagnosis or that the doctor believes them to be imagining the symptoms.

For breathing exercises see pages 71–3.

## *The aims of this chapter*

Some of the effects of overbreathing are bizarre, and often a very frightened person enquires, 'Am I having a stroke? I have this strange tingling in my hands and feet. It's in my mouth, too, my lips are stiff and tingly and my tongue feels too big; it makes it difficult to form some words.'

This chapter explains the symptoms of hyperventilation and suggests some reasons why we have become a nation of hyperventilators. It discusses how the alteration in the acid/alkaline balance of the blood produced by overbreathing can affect the smooth running of every system in the body.

DIY diagnosis can be very dangerous; it is therefore essential to consult your doctor about any medical problems. If you have been told there is nothing wrong and yet are still feeling below par, compare your symptom picture with that of a chronic hyperventilator. If it looks familiar, start working on the practical help

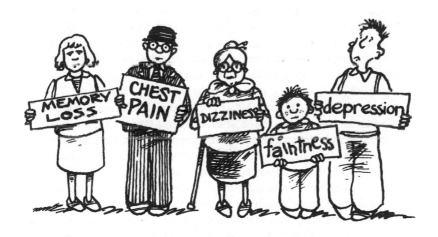

**We're all potential hyperventilators**

programme. Even if you are unsure, try the suggestions. Taking another look at yourself and trying to improve your general health is always worthwhile – nothing is wasted.

## Symptoms of overbreathing

- *Anxiety*
- *Panic attacks*
- *Depression*
- *Feelings of unreality*
- *Sense of hopelessness*
- *Poor memory*
- *Agoraphobia*
- *Other phobias*
- *Palpitations*
- *Shortage of breath.* Inability to take deep breaths. Frequent sighing: 80% of patients who hyperventilate sigh.
- *Dry throat.* Clearing of throat, moistening of dry lips.
- *Dry cough.* Due to water and heat loss from mucosal lining of airway.
- *Stuffy nose.* Dryness, sores in the nose, sniffing, dry lips.
- *Chest pain.* Either a sharp pain lasting seconds or minutes, or a dull ache over the heart and around the breastbone and ribs. This is caused by the strain on the muscles and ligaments by breathing continually from the upper chest. Finger pressure around breastbone or ribs can often find very sore spots. There is also inability to lie on left side. The pain is not usually affected by breathing. It can occur after exercise. Pressure from gas in the stomach can also cause pain. Spasm in coronary artery can cause severe pain and often people arrive at accident and emergency departments (sometimes several times a year) with this. Chest pain does not usually appear with the provocation test.

  Taking a deep breath after relaxing may be an unconscious triggering attack which starts a hyperventilation attack. For this reason I am wary of commercial relaxation tapes which instruct people to take deep breaths.
- *Yawning.* Air hunger.
- *Light-headedness and dizziness* are often the commonest symptoms.

- *Feeling of impending fainting* – all ages.
- *Actual fainting* – more common in the young.
- *Tingling* – hands, feet and around the mouth.
- *Weakness* – in all muscles.
- *Numbness*. Can be anywhere in the body.
- *Jelly legs*. A feeling that the legs cannot support the body.
- *Digestive disturbances* – water brash, bloating, belching, wind in bowel, air swallowing, food intolerances, Irritable Bowel Syndrome.
- *Muscle spasm*. Particularly in the neck and shoulders.
- Claw-like spasm in the hands and feet.
- *Speech difficulties*. Feeling of tongue being swollen.
- *Hallucinations*. Only when symptoms are severe. In order to see 'pictures' a playground game amongst children is to take gulping breaths and be spun round by peers.

### Case studies

James was a sixty-two-year-old retired estate agent. He was a cheerful man and did not seem particularly anxious, although his symptoms were beginning to restrict his activities. He was often light-headed and dizzy and occasionally had fainted. He had undergone full hospital tests including an angiogram (a check to see that the blood supply to the head is not obstructed). All the tests were negative but the symptoms persisted. Often when patients have a long list of symptoms they only relate a few to their doctor because they feel foolish. They usually mention only the ones that cause them most distress, so when James finally said he had difficulty taking a deep breath, had tingling in the hands and around the mouth and also that he was more tired than usual, it was then that the diagnosis of chronic hyperventilation was made. His symptoms disappeared after breathing retraining, and on the occasions when he felt a slight attack coming he was able to ward off the symptoms by bag rebreathing (see page 72–3).

Martin was a hard-working conscientious man of thirty-six. He had never had any anxiety problems and was physically strong. He described his panic attacks as the most bewildering thing that had ever happened to him:

The first one came when I was bending over weeding the garden. My chest felt tight and my heart was beating so strongly that I felt I must be having a heart attack. Everything seemed unreal, the flowers looked so bright and the noise from a lawn mower several gardens away seemed deafening. I was very scared; perspiration was pouring out of me and my arms and legs felt as though they did not belong to me. I made myself walk around and the feelings began to ease although I was still very shaken. My wife later said I was a shade of pale grey. She gave me some sweet tea and this seemed to release an enormous amount of gas from my stomach.

The second one came a few weeks later when I was cleaning the inside of the car. This time I was convinced I had something wrong with my heart and called in the emergency doctor. He said it was just anxiety and suggested a warm bath, some peppermint for the wind and an early night. He seemed to take it so lightly; I was annoyed and far from convinced there was nothing seriously wrong.

I saw my own doctor the next day; he also confirmed there was nothing physically wrong and started to ask questions about my lifestyle. I have to confess I felt annoyed once again, but as he explained things I began to see a pattern; on each occasion I had hurried a big meal then worked in a crouched position. I also had to admit that I had been working longer hours and losing sleep since the baby arrived. It's quite hard to be told to slow down when you're only thirty-six.

Martin's symptoms would suggest that excess gas in the stomach pushed up on his lungs and triggered hyperventilation which caused his panic attacks. In view of the way he had been overtiring himself it is probable that he had been hyperventilating to some degree for some time without noticing it and that this extra trigger was enough to produce the severe symptoms.

Maria felt depressed and hopeless. Her symptoms were numbness, tingling, dizziness, anxiety, palpitations, inability to take a deep breath and a feeling of a lump in her throat. She said she had a continual feeling that something awful was about to happen. A six-week stay in a psychiatric department where she had undergone psychotherapy and been treated with anti-depressants had failed to help her symptoms.

Her story illustrates how the physical symptoms (clearly manifestations of hyperventilation) were discounted. She was fifty-seven years old. Although she had no big life problems she was beginning to feel a gulf between her and the people close to her because of their lack of understanding about her illness.

Her symptoms responded quite quickly to bag rebreathing and this impressed her. She worked hard at her breathing exercises. Her sister participated in her sessions and was also enthusiastic. Within three weeks Maria had greatly reduced her symptoms.

Louise had severe symptoms including blackouts and was understandably very frightened. Her symptoms had been investigated and she was told she was a chronic hyperventilator. Unfortunately she was not given any help and was simply told to slow down her breathing. She did not take this diagnosis seriously and was convinced she was suffering from something much more serious. She continued to feel miserable and to have tingling and numbness around her mouth and in her hands. She lost interest in food because foods that had not upset her in the past began to give her discomfort. Her abdomen would start to swell around mid-afternoon and by evening she would be very bloated and uncomfortable. Her energy levels were low.

Her husband had lost patience with her and felt she was not trying. It was really to please him that she went to an anxiety management group. When she saw others with the same symptoms she was encouraged and soon found that if she used bag rebreathing as soon as the tingling and numbness came she could avoid a blackout. This gave her a lot of confidence. Some people have said that they realize they had the tingling for years before the blackouts developed.

After several months she was still anxious but much improved. Eating without subsequent discomfort was still a problem but otherwise she was leading a normal life.

Julie had never been an anxious person; she enjoyed her

work and had a full social life. She had been to see her doctor because of 'horrible feelings' on waking and at other times during the day. These had come on suddenly. Julie was distressed and very puzzled; she thought she must be developing asthma because she found it difficult to take a good breath. She also complained of dizziness and although she had not actually fainted she often felt she was about to.

Her doctor reassured her she did not have asthma and confirmed she was physically fit. When he asked if she was anxious she denied this. He pointed out that her pulse and breathing were rather rapid for someone who was not feeling anxious. She said her mother had commented several weeks earlier that her breathing was 'funny'. This was about eight weeks after she had cracked two ribs when she slipped by a swimming pool. Her GP had not known about this because she had been on holiday at the time. Things began to make sense now; he concluded that she must have started to overbreathe to avoid the pain and that the habit had persisted when her ribs had healed.

The explanation made sense to her; she started to breathe from her abdomen and joined a yoga class. She controlled daytime symptoms easily with correct breathing, but it took longer for the early morning symptoms to go. She was obviously still sometimes overbreathing in her sleep. She found lying flatter helped (she had used more pillows since the cracked ribs), as did sleeping with the sheet over her face. This gives you back some of the carbon dioxide you are losing.

John was very scared by his first panic attack and wasted no time in seeing a doctor. It was really no surprise to him; he had been waiting for 'something to happen' because on his own admission he had been burning the candle at both ends. He also admitted that he had been dabbling in street drugs for several months – speed and cocaine. He was waiting for a dryer at the launderette when he suddenly felt he could not swallow and was so frightened he thought he would pass out. There had been warning signs over several months but he had ignored them. He had often felt his pulse was racing and his thoughts were jumbled.

He lost all interest in drugs because of the severity of the panic attacks. He took two weeks' rest and ate regular meals. A chest infection complicated his recovery but he eventually did get well.

## Children and hyperventilation

Rapid overbreathing is common in childhood and can be an indication that the child is under severe strain. An American study reviewed the records of thirty-four children under eighteen years of age who had been seen at the Mayo Clinic over a twenty-five-year period. At follow up 40% were still hyperventilating as adults, and many had chronic anxiety and depression problems. Symptoms included headaches, frequent vomiting, irritable bowel, phobias, eye blinking, nail biting and bed wetting.

### Treatment
Professional help should be sought for the child who is hyperventilating unless it is an isolated incident after a cold or fright. A minority of children who hyperventilate hysterically may be using the behaviour to manipulate the adults around them, but in any case this behaviour would need to be investigated and not ignored.

### Breathing retraining for children
This can be made into a game. The paper bag for rebreathing can be coloured with crayons or made into a cartoon character. Singing, playing wind instruments and swimming can also be used to encourage the child to use the lungs fully. It is essential, of course, that the cause of stress in the child's life be investigated. Medical references on hyperventilation follow in the next chapter.

## What can I do about my breathing?

If you cannot get professional help, practise the exercises in the homework section daily. To control a panic attack the breathing is the first avenue to take. The second is to ask yourself when you last ate. The importance of this is described in detail in chapter 6.

37

# 5

# Hyperventilation – Some Medical Evidence

## *History of medical interest in hyperventilation*

Hyperventilation was first documented in 1871 by a man called DaCosta. During the American Civil War he observed 300 soldiers with a strange illness; the men were out of breath, tired, dizzy and complained of palpitations and pain in the chest. They also complained of headaches and disturbed sleep. In spite of all these symptoms DaCosta noted that the men did not have a fever and were otherwise well. The treatment was removal from active duty and rest, but even with this treatment he noted that 'the irritability of the heart remained' and only slowly did it return to normal. DaCosta did not associate these symptoms with overbreathing but he did realize he had seen the same symptoms in his private practice.

The syndrome (collection of symptoms) was called 'DaCosta's Syndrome' or 'Irritable Heart'. It was noticed again in the First World War and was renamed 'Soldiers' Heart' or 'Effort Syndrome'. These terms were rejected by American medical officers in the British Medical Corps because they feared the soldiers would believe they had a heart condition (a great many people who have panic attacks cannot be convinced they have healthy hearts), so this made sense. It was then called 'neuro-circulatory asthenia'. What a convoluted way around finding a name for what could simply have been known as the 'scared soldier syndrome'! Sadly, it seems fighting men were not allowed to feel afraid.

Here is an extract from an article in a medical journal. You should find it very comforting; I have highlighted the really good news. Don't be put off by dates and reference numbers; what is being said is really very exciting:

> It is often assumed that anxiety is the chief or only cause of hyperventilation. On the contrary, any change of mood – happiness, laughter, relief, animated conversation and even

watching television – can frequently be the cause. The first attacks commonly follow a purely physical illness. General anaesthesia and operations are potent triggers. The driving personality, addicted to his work, often develops the first attack at weekends or on holiday. Anxiety then develops out of the persistent symptoms. With repetition the response takes on the character of a conditioned reflex (Cannon 1928).

Although Kerr et al. (1937) had pointed out that the clinical manifestations of anxiety state were produced by hyperventilation, it was Rice (1950) who turned this concept upside down by stating that *patients could be cured by eliminating faulty breathing habits*. Lewis (1964) identified the role of anxiety as a trigger rather than the prime cause. Given habitual hyperventilation, a variety of triggers, psychic or somatic, can initiate the vicious cycle of increased breathing, symptoms, anxiety arising from exacerbating hyperventilation and thus generating more symptoms and more anxiety. *He claimed a 70% cure rate by breathing re-education.* ('Hyperventilation Syndromes in Medicine and Psychiatry: A review', by L. C. Lum, *Journal of the Royal Society of Medicine* 80 (1987), p. 229).

Here is another extract which includes all the familiar symptoms. It is from the *Oxford Textbook of Psychiatry*:

Over-breathing is breathing in a rapid and shallow way which results in a fall of the concentration of carbon dioxide in the blood. The resultant symptoms include dizziness, faintness, numbness and tingling in the hands, feet and face, carpopedal spasms [severe cramp in hands and feet], and precordial discomfort [area of the chest over the heart]. There is also a feeling of breathlessness which may prolong the condition. When a patient has unexplained bodily symptoms, the possibility of persistent overbreathing should always be borne in mind.

The following extract from another article shows that one of the major causes of panic attacks is simply not breathing correctly:

The syndrome (collection of symptoms) characterised by repeated panic attacks has been known by several names including muscular exhaustion of the heart, neurasthenia (nervous exhaustion), irritable heart, anxiety neurosis, effort syndrome, and cardiac neurosis. The manual's definition of panic disorder states that attacks are manifested by the sudden onset of intense apprehension, fear or terror, often associated with feelings of impending doom. The most common symptoms experienced during an attack are dyspnoea [difficulty breathing], choking or smothering sensation, dizziness, vertigo, or unsteady feelings, feelings of unreality, paraesthesias [disordered sensation such as tingling and pins and needles], hot and cold flushes, sweating, faintness, trembling or shaking and fear of dying, doing crazy or doing something uncontrolled during the attack. Attacks usually last minutes; more rarely hours. ('Hyperventilation (shallow breathing) as a Cause of Panic Attacks', by Dr Hibbert, *British Medical Journal* 288 (28.1.1984).)

Research continues into the role of hyperventilation in people with panic disorder. For example, work by Antonio Nardi and colleagues at the Federal University of Rio de Janeiro, Brazil, including studies published in 2003 and 2006, finds that there is growing evidence that they are more sensitive to the effects of hyperventilation.

# 6

## Sugar and Spice and All Things Nice?

### *Hypoglycaemia – low blood sugar*

After the term hypoglycaemia has been explained I will use the term 'unstable blood sugar levels' because this more accurately describes what is about to be discussed. *Hypo* means low, glycaemia means blood sugar, so this term simply means a low level of sugar (glucose) in the blood. *Hyper* means high; therefore hyperglycaemia means a high level of sugar in the blood. Anyone who has low levels of thyroid is said to be *hypo*thyroid. An over-active child is said to be *hyper*active.

You might wonder why there is so much talk of low blood sugar when the greater part of the population eat too much sugar. You could also question why people with two apparently opposite conditions, low blood sugar and diabetes, have similar diets. The person with low blood sugar cuts down on sugar to stop the over-production of insulin. The diabetic cuts down on sugar because his/her body does not produce enough insulin to metabolise the sugar.

#### *Do we need sugar at all?*

We don't need it in the form of sugar; this is empty calories or calories without nutrients. What we do need is complex, unre-fined carbohydrates, whole grains, fruits and vegetables, which are good food value and can also be broken down slowly by the digestive system before being passed into the blood as glucose. When readily available carbohydrate is mentioned it refers to sugar, sweets, white flour and so on; foods that are no sooner in the mouth than, hey presto, they are in the blood. What a jolt this gives the pancreas, the organ which produces the necessary insulin.

## Low blood sugar and the medical profession

Medical interest started in the 1920s, when the American doctor Searle Harris described hypoglycaemia in 1924. Harris noted that hypoglycaemic patients were being misdiagnosed – and inappropriately treated – as neurotic or psychotic. S. Soskin, in the *Journal of Clinical Endocrinology and Metabolism* (1944) states that 'Hyperglycaemia (high blood sugar) does not represent nearly so immediate a threat to the well being of the body as does hypoglycaemia.' That is rather a strong statement, until you consider that a person with diabetes (hyperglycaemia) will be diagnosed and treated correctly whereas the person with hypoglycaemia is unlikely to be correctly diagnosed, can be subjected to countless tests and may be given years of drugs, usually tranquillizers, which worsen the condition. Alternatively, the person may be told they are 'just anxious' or malingering: their symptoms go untreated and they have years of misery.

It cannot be argued that too much insulin does not cause symptoms because the patient who has had stomach surgery or the non-diabetic patient who is given insulin have the same symptom picture as the person with overstimulated nerves who is over-producing insulin.

## There is a lot of it about

Perhaps the truth is that incidence of this condition has risen parallel with many other conditions since the beginning of the century – arthritis, allergies, cancer – but since the symptoms of the latter can be *seen* and treated with drugs or surgery, they are viewed rather differently. Because most of the symptoms of low blood sugar are concerned with the brain (we will see why later), it is easy for medical practitioners to declare that patients are neurotic or fanciful.

The medical profession can be quite blinkered when they don't *expect* the human body to react in a certain way. The case of the benzodiazepines proves this point – the scandal of millions of people worldwide being pharmacologically dependent on tranquillizers like Valium (diazepam), Ativan (lorazepam) and sleeping pills such as temazepam and nitrazepam. They did not see what was under their noses because they did not *expect* it.

## Why is there a lot of it about?

When human beings and medical science become careless about how they treat the human body it is bound to become less efficient and mechanisms that *should* not go wrong, do. What have we done?

- *Changes in diet*
  Think what has happened to our eating patterns this century. From a diet of whole grains, abundant vegetables, meat, poultry, fish and honey we now have an enormous increase in sugar consumption, grains that have had the life knocked out of them and animal products which are contaminated with hormones and antibiotics.

  Whatever happened to the stock pot? It's a long time since a broth of pulses and vegetables was the mainstay of the diet and plates were piled high with greens, baked parsnips, potatoes and carrots. A spoonful of frozen peas as an accompaniment to hamburger or sausage and chips seems to be the norm now.

- *The pace of life*
  People run around in all directions and there is no time to prepare or eat wholesome food. A scant breakfast is followed by a rushed lunch and the family meal is often what a harassed mother can collect in the way of fast food on her way home from work. The time taken to eat it will depend on what is showing on television. Are there many families who talk to each other in a leisurely fashion over wholesome food? You will see later the effect of unhurried well-spaced meals.

- *Prescribed drugs and blood sugar problems*
  If change of diet is the prime cause of low blood sugar problems in modern men and women, then a pill for all ills must be the second. Medical evidence now clearly states that the contraceptive pill, steroids, tranquillizers and sleeping pills, beta blockers and some diuretics (water pills) affect glucose tolerance, cholesterol and triglyceride metabolism. This adverse reaction often goes unnoticed because it is not dramatic. The onset is insidious and often not associated with the drugs either by the doctor or the patient.

• *Increase in the use of non-prescribed drugs*
Alcohol, tobacco, street drugs including heroin, cocaine and cannabis, tea, coffee, and coke all affect blood sugar levels.

### Low blood sugar – shall I go to the doctor?

Unless you feel you have developed low blood sugar symptoms since you have been on a prescribed drug it is probably a waste of time. My experience of the general medical reaction to this problem is: Yes, it is hypoglycaemia – drink sweet tea! or No, only diabetics get that from too much insulin; you are just anxious.

## Does keeping blood sugar levels stable really help?

My belief is that it very definitely does. I have seen hypoglycaemia in a clinical setting on a diabetic ward and also in the community when working with people with anxiety problems. In the latter group, perhaps the condition could more accurately be called unstable blood sugar levels rather than low blood sugar levels because symptoms can occur when the blood sugar levels are within normal limits. It would appear that it is sudden drops which cause the problems rather than the blood sugar level being abnormally low. It is interesting to note that blood sugar levels taken whilst patients were actually having panic attacks were on the lower end of the scale but never actually below normal, and yet their symptoms responded very dramatically to a diet designed to keep the blood sugar levels stable.

After seeing hundreds of people improve, here and in America, when following a low blood sugar eating plan (which needs to be a lot more than just sensible eating), I feel it has a huge part to play in the management not only of anxiety, but also of migraine, premenstrual syndrome (PMS) and some types of asthma. Whilst I see it as an important part of treatment I also feel strongly that the approach to it should be one of common sense.

### Should I have a blood sugar test?

Not unless you have sugar in your urine. The test, called a Glucose Tolerance Test, involves testing blood and urine specimens every half hour for several hours after a measured amount of glucose has been drunk. The test for reasons other than mentioned is not only a waste of time, but can also make the patient feel very unwell for several days.

I see the answer as very simple: if the symptoms are coming from unstable blood sugar levels they will respond to diet within a few days; if they do not, then it is not a blood sugar problem.

In my work in the community over several years it has been a great joy to see so many 'no breakfast, sandwich lunch, large evening meal' eaters reduce their adrenaline levels, lose so many of their anxiety symptoms, and become confident and in charge by simply stopping their blood sugar levels from rapidly bouncing up and down. I have called this 'kangarooing' in an attempt to give clients an image of what they are doing to themselves.

### It's your body

I never cease to marvel at the accuracy of people's intuitive feelings about what ails their bodies. If you feel your symptom picture fits with the symptoms below follow the recommendations; you have nothing to lose. Do remember the condition brought about by unstable blood sugar levels is not an illness, it is merely a result of stress and incorrect diet.

## Symptoms of unstable blood sugar levels

Many of the anxiety symptoms discussed in the preceding chapters also appear when the blood sugar drops quickly so I will not cover them again in detail. You should be very familiar with the symptoms by now.

We have seen that when the body is under stress the circulation is affected and the result is palpitations, missed heart beats and so on. In addition to the expected symptoms there are some which are more specific to changing blood sugar levels. These are dull headaches, inner trembling but no visible shaking, sugar craving, waking between 3 a.m. and 5 a.m. alert, anxious and sometimes very hungry, low energy mid-morning and mid-afternoon, twitching eyelid muscles, wanting to eat again about an hour after the evening meal, no desire for breakfast, lapses in concentration, tenderness over the pancreas and sore trigger points over the left lower ribs.

### Adrenal exhaustion – nervous exhaustion

As has been said, when the blood sugar drops the adrenal glands above the kidneys produce cortisone and adrenaline to make the stored glucose available for use. When these glands are continually harassed the condition known as adrenal exhaustion follows; the body is no longer able to deal with stress. Anxiety, panic attacks, depression, irritability and eventual change of personality can arise from the nerve cells being deprived of nourishment.

### Unstable blood sugar levels and panic attacks

You will now understand why a dramatic drop in blood sugar levels causes a flood of adrenaline. Why this is such a potent trigger for a panic attack is explained on page 48.

### Caution – pay attention!

Workers and clients alike have confessed they have skipped the chapter on blood sugar levels in my books thinking I was just vaguely talking about nutrition. It was not until they heard me teach (or perhaps preach would be a better word) that they got the full implication of the subject. When people fully understand the mechanism involved and just how their neglect is hurting their nervous system they are much more willing to follow the rules.

## What happens when I don't eat properly

Sugar is an important constituent of the body. In the form of glucose it gets into the bloodstream from the food we eat. The excess is stored in the liver as glycogen and it is on this store that we call when there is no food left in the digestive tract. We do *not* need large quantities of sugar to keep this supply of glucose steady because most foods, with the exception of fats, can be turned into glucose. Proteins (meat, fish, dairy produce, nuts, seeds, pulses) are converted by the liver into glucose but this only happens when the bowel is empty of carbohydrate (sugar, bread, cakes, biscuits, cereals, fruit and vegetables).

### Brain food

Glucose can be considered the fuel of the body. The brain is totally dependent on this form of food – without it, it would die. It is important to remember this when looking at the list of symptoms caused by unstable blood sugar levels. The brain cannot utilize other foods such as protein the way tissues like the muscles can; this is why there are so many symptoms of altered brain chemistry when the blood sugar level drops quickly. Another point to remember is that the brain deprived of glucose is also deprived of oxygen. Have you noticed how you yawn when you go too long without food? Poor availability of glucose to the brain can also cause many of the symptoms associated with this condition, without the blood sugar level being low at all. If the circulation to the head were affected, say, by tension in the neck and shoulders the brain cells are bound to be half starved because the blood carries the glucose. You will see later how this can cause migraine.

### How is the blood sugar regulated?

When food is eaten, the pancreas, an organ on the left side of the body near the stomach, pours out regulated amounts of a hormone called insulin. If this organ is working properly and if food intake is adequate then all is well.

### What can go wrong with this system?

Two things: either the pancreas can fail and not produce enough insulin which results in DIABETES – HYPERGLYCAEMIA; or the pancreas can be hyperactive and produce too much insulin, resulting in LOW BLOOD SUGAR – HYPOGLYCAEMIA.

### Why does the pancreas overwork?

Because it gets the wrong messages. When you are in a nervous state all the nerves are overstimulated. This includes the nerves to the pancreas. So it is being told: go faster, go faster, and it throws out more and more insulin – much more than the body requires. The result is that the available glucose is quickly used and the blood sugar levels drop dramatically.

### Common reasons why the pancreas is overstimulated

• *Extra demands*: Exercise, stress, pregnancy, the premenstrual phase, the effects of some drugs.

- *Rarer reasons*: Glucose sensitivity, under-function of the pituitary, thyroid or adrenal glands, liver disease, disease of the pancreas.

## *Why does a drop in blood sugar make me feel so awful?*

- When your brain is starved, it begins to do strange things.
- When there is no food left and the blood sugar is low, the stomach sends a message to the brain saying HELP! I'm hungry! What are you going to do?

### *The brain replies*

Don't worry, I will get you some food (glucose) out of the larder (the liver), but in order to unlock the larder door I have to send a messenger with a key. This chemical messenger is a spurt of adrenaline. The good news is, when the messenger opens the door, glucose will be released and you can keep going; the bad news is you have already seen too much of this messenger because other systems in your body (breathing, muscles) are not working well since your nerves have been in trouble, and the adrenaline brings all the symptoms you dread most: panic, shaking, palpitations, agoraphobia and so on. Are you beginning to see why it is so important to eat correctly?

### *Are some people reluctant to change their eating habits?*

One worker asked whether it wasn't stressful to have to keep to a diet, when someone was already having difficulty coping. My reply was yes, some people had grumbled quite a lot, but it was pointed out to them that it was a small price to pay for reduced anxiety feelings and the control of panic attacks. My experience is that people soon feel the benefit and become very enthusiastic. There are also those who become overconfident and after a few symptom-free weeks descend to their old eating habits. It usually takes only one panic attack to send them rushing back to the book.

### *Can the effects of diet lapses be delayed?*

Yes. What you sow one day you may not reap until the next. It was fascinating to watch a large group of people have a return of symptoms when they digressed. Panic attacks abounded on Monday mornings (no, it was not the washing). This happened when the normal evening meal was replaced by Sunday tea with mother. Large quantities of bread, cakes and biscuits would throw the blood sugar levels into confusion and the result would be a panic attack. The regular Saturday morning panic attack proved to be alcohol induced. Even a small quantity is enough to provoke symptoms if the blood sugar levels are unstable. This makes sense because the main misery of a hangover is hypoglycaemia. People are able to accept that they can precipitate a panic attack by missing a meal but find it harder to accept that eating the wrong foods can do the same.

### Do I risk more than exhausted nerves?

Yes, you do. There is a great deal of evidence to show that people who constantly strain their bodies by kangarooing blood sugar levels run a greater risk of developing chronic conditions such as diabetes, arthritis, allergies, migraine, asthma, obesity, blackouts and epilepsy.

### Why do unstable blood sugar levels upset my digestion?

When insulin is overproduced it stimulates the stomach which in turn increases the flow of digestive secretions. An over-acid stomach results and can cause heartburn, indigestion, food allergies and hiatus hernia.

### Why do unstable blood sugar levels trigger migraine?

Many migraine sufferers associate symptoms of irritability and headaches if they miss meals. The City of London Migraine Clinic has published several leaflets on this (see Useful Addresses).

As the blood sugar falls, more blood is pumped to the brain to prevent the level of glucose becoming dangerously low. This causes pressure on the cranial nerves. These nerves serve more than the head; that is why there are apparently unrelated symptoms. For example, when the nerves to the stomach or liver are involved symptoms such as diarrhoea can occur, or if it were the nerve to the arm affected there could be tingling or numbness. If the increased pressure affects the nerves to the ears, hypersensitivity to sound or tinnitus (ringing in the ears) can result. It is easy to see why visual disturbances, such as difficulty focusing, flashing lights, partial loss of vision, sensitivity to light and bloodshot eyes, are so often reported in migraine sufferers. Food sensitivities affect the blood glucose levels; it follows therefore that they can also trigger migraines.

### Can unstable blood sugar levels cause aching joints and muscles?

Yes they can. When the adrenal glands are exhausted cortisone production is lowered. This important hormone is necessary not only for the control of stress, but also for the metabolism of carbohydrate. The other vital function of cortisone is to protect the body from inflammation. This can be confirmed by how dramatically treatment with cortisone and other steroids can reduce the pain of arthritis. So whilst at first it might sound a little far-fetched to say if you don't eat sensibly you could risk aches and pains, when you consider the role of cortisone and how its output diminishes when the blood sugar is low, then the connection becomes clearer.

The fact that rheumatoid arthritis often clears up during pregnancy also confirms this. At this time the increase in pituitary (the so-called master gland of the body) hormones and cortisone work to counteract the effect of insulin. Therefore if the insulin production is lowered the blood sugar will not be jumping all over the place; it will remain stable.

### Premenstrual syndrome and unstable blood sugar levels

More and more pieces of the jigsaw fit together when the part that hormones play is understood. To go back to the over-acid stomach again, this does not absorb calcium efficiently. Nerves need calcium to function properly. Reduced levels lead to hypersensitivity and irritability of the nervous system. The frayed nerves, muscle cramps and fluid retention of premenstrual tension can all be attributed to this and an imbalance of the sodium and potassium levels. It is uncomfortable for the body to be swollen with fluid but even more so when the brain is waterlogged. Severe headaches, rapid mood swings and outbursts of rage are distressingly common symptoms. The premenstrual craving for sweets, chocolates and other carbohydrates is a sign that all is not well with the blood sugar levels. More about PMS on pages 44 and 52.

*Will I get diabetes if I ignore unstable blood sugar levels?*

No, not necessarily, but you do run a risk, particularly if you gain a lot of weight, or are from a family where there is a history of diabetes or other conditions associated with low blood sugar. A pancreas which is working to death dealing with a high refined carbohydrate diet and long gaps between meals does often give up trying.

*What other conditions are associated with unstable blood sugar levels?*

Whilst some physicians do not believe that low blood sugar levels have any connection with the development of chronic illness, others are firmly convinced that sustained unstable blood sugar levels precede many illnesses, and that improvement or cure can be gained by simply following a low blood sugar eating plan. A great deal of work has been done on this in America (see Further Reading). Here are some of the conditions implicated:

| | | |
|---|---|---|
| obesity | fainting | allergies |
| hyperactivity | blackouts | migraine |
| anxiety | facial pain | stomach ulcers |
| depression | epilepsy | addictions |
| asthma | arthritis | tinnitus |
| loss of interest in sex | | |

There is no need to be alarmed by this list; eating sensibly avoids low blood sugar.

*Must I eat like this for ever?*

No. Don't worry, as your nerves get stronger and your pancreas stops working overtime you can have treats. You can add all your old favourites to a sensible diet. There is no need to make a big issue of it.

*Case histories*

During the years I ran a tranquillizer withdrawal support group there were several young women and two young men who had no drug history at all who came for help with panic attacks. The women had all been trying to lose weight on crash diets or by missing meals, and both the young men had altered their diets for vigorous exercise. One had been eating steak and eggs one day and Mars bars the next. When they resumed healthy eating the panic attacks vanished. If you are overweight the Weight Watchers' flexible diet takes care of losing weight and unstable blood sugar levels. The support is also very valuable. They are usually in the local paper or Yellow Pages. The Rosemary Conley approach to weight loss is also very popular. Her book *New Inch Loss Plan* describes a diet that is very easy to keep to even if you are cooking for others (see Further Reading, page 113).

John, a thirty-four-year-old teacher, had been having migraine attacks since he was in the sixth form (this was also when he started smoking). He remembered that smoking had curbed his appetite somewhat and he stopped having breakfast. He was eventually prescribed tranquillizers because the migraines were attributed to a stressful job. They did not help and he continued to have regular one-sided blinding headaches which often resulted in vomiting. As he withdrew from tranquillizers he ate regular balanced meals, cut down his smoking and never smoked without eating. He was astonished by how this helped the headaches.

Suzie was twenty-eight and had suffered severe premenstrual syndrome for three years. She was depressed and very frightened by the panic attacks and feelings of rage. Her husband was supportive but they were both very concerned about the effect her behaviour was having on their young family. For almost half the month she felt bloated, irritable and clumsy. She dropped things and could not knit. Her husband noticed her hands and face were swollen during the premenstrual phase. He felt this was because she ate so much chocolate when her period was due. She agreed this was so and she also complained of constipation, a swollen abdomen and leg cramps. These were so bad they woke her in the night. After three months on a balanced diet and supplements (see pages 75–7) she lost a stone in weight and apart from still being a bit 'ratty' premenstrually she lost all her symptoms.

# 7

## Panic Attacks and Drugs

Any substance which *sedates* (calms the nervous system), be it alcohol, prescribed drugs or street drugs, can be a cause of panic attacks. When the adrenaline levels are artificially reduced by the drugs it is like putting a lid on a volcano. When the lid is taken off – withdrawal – adrenaline rushes out with even greater force and then all the terrible feelings of panic, palpitations, sweating and so on occur.

### *Can tranquillizers and sleeping pills cause panic attacks?*

Yes they can. Side effects and withdrawal effects can both cause panic attacks. This is confusing and has caused a great deal of distress – the very drugs which are supposed to stop panic attacks, can, in some people, actually *cause* them. It is now well documented that these drugs, known as the benzodiazepines, can produce anxiety symptoms at the beginning of therapy. This might be in a person who had no anxiety symptoms prior to treatment – perhaps someone prescribed diazepam for muscle spasm. This is called the paradoxical reaction. Withdrawal of the drugs can also cause great problems and therefore must be done slowly with supervision. During withdrawal, anxiety levels can be six times greater than the pre-drug levels, even in people who have been given identical tablets and have no knowledge that their drugs are being withdrawn. It is, therefore, not a matter of 'Oh dear, I haven't had my Valium today, I'm going to feel awful'. With anxiety levels sky-high panic attacks abound.

### *Can withdrawal symptoms appear when I'm still taking the pills?*

Yes. This is an important point to consider. It is because the body has become used to them and the withdrawal symptoms are the body's demand for more. You can have panic attacks between doses. The drugs involved are listed below but for full information on the side effects, withdrawal reactions and a complete withdrawal programme, read *Tranquillizers and Antidepressants: When to take them, how to stop*, by Professor Malcolm Lader (Sheldon Press).

| Chemical name | Brand name |
|---|---|
| Diazepam | Valium |
| Lorazepam | Ativan |
| Chlordiazepoxide | Librium |
| Temazepam | Normison, Euhypnos |
| Oxazepam | Serenid |
| Nitrazepam | Mogadon |
| Clobazam* | Frisium* |

\* Not prescribed for anxiety

Here are some guidelines for professionals in case you need information for your doctor. Do remember you must not stop any prescribed drugs without consulting your doctor, and also be reassured that if you come off slowly and take care of yourself you can recover completely; countless numbers have.

# Guidelines

From: *Current Problems* (Committee on Safety of Medicines), Number 21, January 1988 (in 2005 this Committee merged with another body to become the Commission on Human Medicines)

### Benzodiazepines, Dependence and Withdrawal Symptoms

There has been concern for many years regarding benzodiazepine dependence (*British Medical Journal* 1980, 910–912). Such dependence is becoming increasingly worrying.

Withdrawal symptoms include anxiety, tremor, confusion, insomnia, perception disorders, fits, depression, gastrointestinal and other somatic symptoms. These may sometimes be difficult to distinguish from the symptoms of the original illness.

It is important to note that withdrawal symptoms can occur with benzodiazepines following therapeutic doses given for short periods of time.

Withdrawal effects usually appear shortly after stopping a

benzodiazepine with a short half-life. Symptoms may continue for weeks or months. No epidemiological evidence is available to suggest that one benzodiazepine is more responsible for the development of dependency or withdrawal symptoms than another. The Committee on Safety of Medicines recommends that the use of benzodiazepines should be limited in the following ways.

## Uses

### As anxiolytics

(1) Benzodiazepines are indicated for the short-term relief (two to four weeks only) of anxiety that is severe, disabling or subjecting the individual to unacceptable distress, occurring alone or in association with insomnia or short-term psychosomatic organic or psychotic illness.

(2) The use of benzodiazepines to treat short-term 'mild' anxiety is inappropriate and unsuitable.

### As hypnotics [sleep-inducing drugs]

(3) Benzodiazepines should be used to treat insomnia only when it is severe, disabling, or subjecting the individual to extreme distress.

## Dose

(1) The lowest dose which can control the symptoms should be used. It should not be continued beyond four weeks.

(2) Long-term chronic use is not recommended.

(3) Treatment should always be tapered off gradually.

(4) Patients who have taken benzodiazepines for a long time may require a longer period during which doses are reduced.

(5) When a benzodiazepine is used as a hypnotic, treatment should, if possible, be intermittent.

## Precautions

(1) Benzodiazepines should not be used alone to treat depression or anxiety associated with depression. Suicide may be precipitated in such patients.

(2) They should not be used for phobic or obsessional states.

(3) They should not be used for the treatment of chronic psychosis.

(4) In case of loss or bereavement, psychological adjustment may be inhibited by benzodiazepines.
(5) Disinhibiting effects may be manifested in various ways. Suicide may be precipitated in patients who are depressed, and aggressive behaviour towards self and others may be precipitated. Extreme caution should therefore be used in prescribing benzodiazepines in patients with personality disorders.

### Can antidepressants cause panic attacks?

Yes. Although it is less widely acknowledged it is nevertheless true. Antidepressants can be very useful drugs and dramatically help some people but anyone who has worked with large numbers of people on antidepressants cannot fail to observe that they also, at the beginning of therapy, can make the patient very anxious, and for some people there is a very well-defined withdrawal syndrome with rebound anxiety and rebound depression when the drugs are stopped. This is helped by gradual withdrawal. The patient is often told these drugs won't help the depression for several weeks; they are rarely told they could feel more anxious at first, but it will pass. This is one of the main reasons why people discontinue taking them after a few days. The drug Prozac has been in the news over the years. For some it has been a magical relief from depression; for others it caused unbearable anxiety symptoms. Antidepressant drugs include:

Prothiaden (dothiepin/dosulepin)
Amitriptyline
Fluanxol
Triptaphen

### Do any other prescribed drugs cause panic attacks?

Yes: drugs which are not prescribed for anxiety but have a sedative action as a side effect. These include: antihistamines, cimetidine (Tagamet), beta blockers and, strangely enough, some antibiotics. For many years now people have been reporting psychological symptoms when they were on or coming off antibiotics. This has largely been considered fanciful until recently when research has

shown that some antibiotics share the same receptors in the brain
as tranquillizers.

## Cigarettes and panic attacks

Nicotine is a pernicious addiction because it both sedates and
stimulates. A person may smoke a cigarette to calm their nerves
but if the same person smoked before a meal or smoked too much
they could become very jittery or even have a panic attack. Panic
attacks in cigarette withdrawal have been mentioned in the medical
literature and it is worth noting that they may not appear for some
months after complete withdrawal. Don't use this as an excuse for
continuing to smoke! They are transient. The other point worth
noting is that if you cut down your smoking by more than a third
at one time you can experience a full-blown withdrawal effect.
But having said that, some people don't have any symptoms at
all when they stop; others experience only the craving. For those
who experience severe physical and emotional symptoms, a word
of comfort. This has much more to do with your biochemistry
than with your lack of will-power. It is possibly because of this,
and also the masked allergy factor, that some people find giving
up so difficult. A hidden or masked allergy can happen with *any*
substance which is taken into the body daily; when the body is
denied the substance then the symptoms appear.

### Do you panic because you are still smoking?

Some people worry a great deal about being dependent on nicotine but fail repeatedly in their attempts to stop. These people are
often scorned by those who claim it is only will-power that is
required. Will-power certainly comes into it; for the physically
addicted/allergic smoker, there is a lot more to it – lack of will-
power or weakness cannot be the cause of swollen joints or skin
problems, and so on.

### Severe nicotine withdrawal

For some people there is a clearly defined withdrawal syndrome
(a collection of symptoms) when they abstain from nicotine. This
is not surprising because the drug affects many systems in the

body and it is just like giving up heroin, tranquillizers or any other addictive substance. Common complaints are:

* feeling anxious and depressed
* panic attacks
* irritability
* headaches
* confused thoughts
* constipation
* sugar craving
* coffee craving
* aching joints and muscles.

People who have tried several times to stop smoking know these feelings very well; they even know which symptoms will come in the first week and how long it takes for the joint pains to start, and so on. Unfortunately, they also know how quickly the symptoms go when they resume smoking.

There are a number of reasons for repeated failure to give up smoking. Lack of information heads the list; if people know what to expect and are reassured that the feelings will not last for ever they stand a much better chance of succeeding. Also if they prepare their bodies for the trauma (make no mistake, it can take its toll physically), the chances of success are further improved.

### Are you in this trap?

If you are an addictive smoker you are likely to have unstable blood sugar levels. Read chapter 6 carefully and adjust your diet accordingly. **If your blood sugar is allowed to drop you are ten times more likely to beg someone for a cigarette**. Keep a bag of sunflower seeds in your pocket and at first eat some every hour between meals. They are full of good things and will keep your blood sugar levels stable. Another way in which diet can help you is to eat foods which leave an alkaline residue, or ash, when they are broken down in the body; vegetables, particularly raw vegetables, and the less sweet fruits are good. Research has shown an over-acid body is more likely to crave cigarettes.

## *You need more than a good diet*

Many people are now seeking natural ways to cleanse the digestive system from the effects of drugs and careless eating habits and also to build up the nervous system and immune system with supplements of vitamins and minerals. Take an honest look at your nutritional state and build your body up for the coming stress. Every cigarette you smoke robs you of 25 mgms of vitamin C, so you are bound to be short of this. Also your requirements for this and all nutrients rises sharply when your body is under siege. Taking large quantities of certain nutrients is not very helpful since they often depend upon each other for absorption. One way around this is to take both a good quality multivitamin and multimineral preparation, and if you feel you can identify any particular deficiency you can take an additional supply of that mineral or vitamin.

There are other helpful supplements, Vitamin C and magnesium both help to rid the body of poisons. Vitamin C strengthens the immune system and eases withdrawal symptoms. Vitamin B3, niacin, has also been found to be helpful. This chemical, which can also be bought in the form known as nicotinic acid, is similar in structure to nicotine. Niacin is thought to resemble the endogenous benzodiazepine, that is, a tranquillizing substance similar to diazepam (Valium) made in the brain. The usual recommended dose is to build up to 100 mgms morning and 100 mgms at night. Don't be surprised if your skin pricks and you look like a beetroot twenty minutes or so after taking it. It is a harmless flush and is beneficial; it improves circulation to the extremities (it is used for chilblains and Raynaud's Disease, a condition characterized by cold, white or blue fingers, caused by spasm in the arteries in the hands) and acts like an internal sauna. It is also known to be essential to the health of the bowel. People who are always cold often find this supplement helpful and many people say that after the first few doses they feel very much calmer. To avoid the flush you could ask for niacinimide, another form of vitamin B3. The only thing to remember is to take all the B vitamins if you take this. No B vitamins should be taken in isolation because it depletes the store of the others.

It is essential to have expert advice on nutrition in general, and Penny Davenport, who runs New Nutrition at the Healthy Living Clinic in Battle, West Sussex, is an experienced nutritionist who can provide leaflets, information and advice (see Useful Addresses).

## Caffeine and panic attacks

So many people drink endless cups of tea and coffee each day and then wonder why they are nervous. A cup of strong tea or coffee on an empty stomach is a potent trigger for panic attacks. Most people don't think of caffeine as a drug, or realize it can affect more than the nervous system. Make an effort to cut down, particularly if you have sore breasts, allergies, digestive problems, cystitis or the restless legs syndrome; that awful feeling also known as 'singing legs' when your legs won't relax and you feel the need to move them even when you are in bed. You might have no trouble at all in giving up tea and coffee completely for a while, or even for good, but it is important to note that some people do experience great difficulties when they attempt this, and strangely enough it is not always people who are heavy tea, coffee or coke drinkers who suffer. In susceptible people, cutting down on caffeine can bring lethargy, and total abstinence can result in nausea, severe headache, muscle and joint pains and depression.

### A blinding headache

'The caffeine storm' develops when, during withdrawal, all the caffeine which has been stored in the body is released into the bloodstream, and in effect causes a form of caffeine poisoning. The resulting headache is particularly severe, and in fact caffeine addicts are used to test the efficacy of headache drugs. Typically, as soon as tea or coffee is taken, even in a small amount, the headache eases, but the same cannot be said for the depression which often accompanies caffeine withdrawal. Some people feel down for several days. Occasionally after complete withdrawal, the depression can last for months. Homoeopathic treatment for caffeine addiction can be helpful or mild symptoms can often be relieved by putting a grain of coffee or a couple of drops of tea under the tongue. The above information is not meant to discourage you from cleaning some of the caffeine out of your system; on the contrary, your bowel, kidneys and nervous system would welcome this. It has been included to help you to understand that some of the everyday things we drink are powerful drugs and some people will experience drug withdrawal symptoms; cut down slowly if you are one of the unlucky ones. You can do this by mixing decaffeinated coffee with your usual blend then increasing the amount of it until you are drinking all decaffeinated. Choose a brand that has not used chemicals for the decaffeination process. You might choose to take smaller quantities of weak filter coffee; this way you get fewer solids.

## Street drugs and panic attacks

All the illegal drugs can cause panic attacks. Those who take LSD, speed (amphetamines) and cocaine, and users who mix street drugs and the benzodiazepines (tranquillizers and sleeping pills) are most at risk. Many young people who use cannabis see it as an innocuous substance. This is far from the truth. It can cause serious psychological problems including nervous breakdown, and it is also very common for regular users to suffer panic attacks and depression during withdrawal.

## Jet lag and panic attacks

This has nothing to do with fear of flying. It happens after the journey, usually for about a week. Typically, these attacks take the form of mild panic attacks on waking, but they can occur at other times during the day. They may be a result of the blood sugar levels being disturbed by eating against the body clock, or they may be due to increased levels of a brain chemical called serotonin. This results in serotonin irritation syndrome. The air around us is charged negatively and positively. When there is an excess of positive ions, animals have been shown to become restless, irritable and anxious. It affects sensitive humans too, usually weather-sensitive people. Have you ever felt swollen, too tight for your skin, headachey with a stuffy nose before a storm, when there was a warm wind, at the full moon, or when you were in an office full of computer screens and fluorescent lights? You could also feel anxious or depressed: 'under the weather'.

A small machine which produces negative ions is the answer. These are available in most department stores and cost from £20. They are also very helpful for people with allergies or chest problems. Negative ions are also produced by running water (even the shower) and at the sea. For more information on this see Further Reading (page 113). See also pages 104–5.

# PART TWO
# Helping Yourself

# 8

## Improve Your Breathing

### *Choose to live – B-R-E-A-T-H-E*

Life is breath. It is the most important function of the body. We may be able to fast, or even go without fluid for a while, but we cannot stop breathing for more than a few minutes. So it must be the most important of the bodily functions.

Correct breathing has a profound effect on the nervous system, clear thinking and even on the spiritual life. Careless breathing will shorten our lifespan and predispose us to a great many diseases, not only diseases of the respiratory system but of every system of the body.

#### *Why have we developed poor breathing habits?*

'Civilized' human beings have developed tense attitudes in walking, sitting and standing; the shoulders are raised, the chest narrowed and the head pulled back. This does not allow us to use our full lung capacity. Animals, 'primitive' people and children do not have this problem.

#### *Breath holding*

Do you hold your breath? Wilhelm Reich, a psychoanalyst famous in the 40s and 50s, noticed that many of his patients held their breath and delayed breathing out to control their feelings. This would serve to slow down the metabolic rate (the rate at which they would burn up their food) which would reduce the flow of adrenaline and help to control feelings of anxiety.

### *Control your breath, control your life*

The amount of energy you have will be in proportion to the way you breathe. When you inhale you are taking in more than the constituents of air, you are also taking in the life force (*prana*, universal energy, *chi*). You will not find reference to this in Gray's *Anatomy* but that does not mean it does not exist. In the

West we are just beginning to see what our Eastern brothers and sisters have been aware of for thousands of years, but progress is slow because of lack of 'evidence'. It does not leave a chemical residue and it is difficult to measure this energy in conventional terms. We have a lot to learn. The life force is there for the taking; are you utilizing it?

### How is this energy used?

*Prana* is taken in by the nervous system and gives strength and vitality – hence the *vital force* (another name it is known by). This energy is used and needs replenishing in the same way that there has to be a continual supply of oxygen and food for the needs of the body. If the supply of *prana* is not enough the person becomes devitalized and we speak of the sufferer having low energy, run-down batteries, or of them being drained. For a healthy body, not only has the supply of *prana* to be adequate, but it must also have free access to all parts of the body.

### What causes blocks in the flow of prana?

Bad breathing, tension, injury, bad posture, disease, worry, sending negative thought patterns to parts of the body, all cause blocks.

If you become 'blocked' you can help yourself by using breathing exercises, stretching exercises, meditation, relaxation, and yoga. There are also opportunities for professional help. Most recognized alternative therapies increase the supply and regulate the flow of *prana*. They include: acupuncture, acupressure, shiatsu, yoga, t'ai chi, massage, homoeopathy, aromatherapy, reflexology, and therapeutic touch. Therapeutic tough is explained on pages 106–8.

## Start breathing today

Controlled breathing can put you in charge of every aspect of your life, not only to improve your physical health but also to bring mastery over fear and other unwanted emotions such as anger and jealousy. Learning the science of breath is the most important contribution you can make to improving your life.

**Respiratory system**

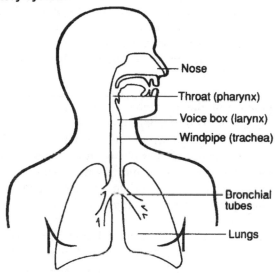

## What do we breathe with?

The lungs, two spongy sacs, and the air passages leading to them. The air passages are the nose, the throat (pharynx), the voice box (larynx), the windpipe (trachea) and the bronchial tubes. These together make up the respiratory system (shown above).

### Some questions about breathing

- *Mouth or nose breathing?*
  When we breathe in through the nose air is warmed and germs and other impurities are filtered out. When we breathe in through the mouth this does not happen. The result is a parched tongue, dry throat and often a cough. You must have noticed this when you have a blocked nose.
- *How does the air get into the lungs?*
  The strong, sheet-like muscle called the diaphragm which separates the chest from the abdomen draws the air into the lungs.
- *Can I control the action of this muscle?*
  This is an important point. Although the action of the diaphragm is automatic like the action of the heart, *it can come*

67

*under the control of the will.* This is the first thing you need to know when you start to retrain your breathing. Whilst this muscle will function and not let you down, if you give it lazy messages and imprison it with tension, it can become very dull. When it expands, the capacity of the lungs is increased and the air rushes in. When it relaxes the air is pushed out.

- *How does poor breathing affect circulation?*
Blood pumped by the heart goes via the arteries to tiny tubes called capillaries. This reaches and nourishes every part of the body. It is bright red and full of vital nutrients. When it returns in veins to the heart, dull and poisoned by the waste products of metabolism (the process of burning the food we eat), it then goes to the lungs where a clean-up operation begins. The success of that operation depends on *how you breathe.*

- *Have you got dirty blood?*
Good breathing will result in clean blood being poured back into the system. Poor breathing will result in dirty blood being returned to the system. It's rather like using the same dirty bathwater over and over again. Would you do that to your skin?

- *Have you got clean blood?*
When blood is properly exposed to the air in the lungs it is not only cleaned but also takes up the oxygen needed to nourish the whole body. This is essential for all systems but particularly for the digestion; poor digestion and hyperventilation often go together. Insufficient oxygen means poor absorption of food, poor elimination of waste and chronic vague ill health. Are you going to choose health? Are you going to breathe?

## Types of breathing

- *Collar bone or shoulder breathing (hyperventilation)*
This is the worst type of breathing; it is positively dangerous. It fills only the upper portion of the lungs.
- *Rib or mid breathing*
This is marginally better, but not good enough. This fills the middle of the lungs and covers a larger area.
- *Low, diaphragmatic and abdominal breathing*
This is a great improvement; the lungs are given much more space and more air can be inhaled.

- *The complete or full breath*
  This is an excellent way to breathe; all the breathing tools we have been given are used. There is plenty of movement in the whole chest. All the air cells and all the breathing muscles, including the muscles between the ribs, are used. When the diaphragm expands and the ribs are pushed out the lungs have room to inflate. If you don't move these muscles it's like trying to inflate a balloon inside a small box.

**The three portions of the lung used in breathing**

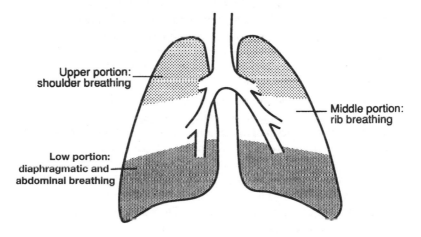

Upper portion: shoulder breathing

Middle portion: rib breathing

Low portion: diaphragmatic and abdominal breathing

## *Treat yourself – take a full breath*

Imagine that your chest has three sections and each one is a coloured balloon:

A.  Shoulder balloon is blue
B.  Rib balloon is green
C.  Diaphragm and abdomen balloon is yellow.

### *Becoming aware of the three sections*

A.  Stand or sit with a straight back and breathe into the blue balloon; lift your shoulders towards your ears and breathe in. Notice what it feels like to inflate the top part of your lungs.

    [*Relax*]

B.  In the same position, push out the chest and ribs and breathe into the green balloon. Be aware of how different that feels.

[*Relax*]

C.  Breathe into the yellow balloon by pushing the front wall of your abdomen, above your navel, slightly down and out and notice how much space you are making inside. You will feel the tension in the gut release as you do this.

[*Relax*]

Imagine the balloons are in boxes and that when you use your muscles you are opening the boxes to allow the balloons to fill with air. A complete breath is impossible if the balloons are imprisoned.

### *Using the complete breath*

By now you should be aware of these three distinct 'boxes'. Bringing the breath into all three in a flowing rhythmic movement is the secret of the complete breath. The movements are not jerky or vigorous, they are slow and peaceful. Be patient when you practise, it is not easy. The results are well worth it so do work for at least two fifteen-minute sessions per day. If you are the type of person who won't take special time for your health, you could build the exercises into daily living; while you wait for the kettle to boil, when you're in the queue for the bathroom or when you take a short stroll at lunchtime to get out of the stale air of the office. There is no need at this stage to count how many breaths you take per minute because your breathing will naturally be slowed; it takes much longer to use the abdomen, chest and shoulders to breathe, rather than just breathing from the shoulders.

*As you breathe in:*
- lift the diaphragm;
- expand the chest and ribs;
- slightly lift the shoulders.

*As you breathe out:*
- let your shoulders fall;
- let your ribs sink back;
- pull the tummy in and then gently up to push out the last of the air.

70

### Are some people afraid to change their breathing?

Yes. Many people are nervous about this. Perhaps it is because when they have tried they feel light-headed or breathless. This is because they have changed the levels of carbon dioxide in the blood too quickly and they have brought on the very symptoms they fear. This illustrates just how unhealthy their breathing is, and they need to have a rest and start again, going at the right speed for them. They also need to be reassured that if they persevere the light-headedness will go and a feeling of relaxation will take over. If you have been breathing rapidly from the upper chest it is unrealistic to try to breathe eight times a minute at your first attempt. Change the rate and depth of your breathing in stages. Perhaps you would be better to master abdominal breathing first. It is not quite as good but still very helpful. It also needs less concentration so can be done whilst you are walking around or working.

### Become aware of how you are breathing

It will take time for better breathing habits to become automatic, so be patient with yourself. To gauge how many times per minute you are breathing look at a watch or clock when you have been at rest for a few minutes and count how many times you breathe in and out (this is one breath) in thirty seconds. Double this and you have your respiration rate per minute. If it is sixteen or more you would be wise to follow the exercise below. If you find it difficult to count your breaths, ask a family member to do it when you are not aware of what they are doing.

#### Exercise

You might find the following exercises boring, but the results will be worth it. Some people have difficulty raising the abdomen. It can help to place a warm, covered hot water bottle on your tummy; it can help to relax you and also gives you a little weight to lift. Some people find lying on the tummy easier; the resistance of the floor helps.

1. Place one hand on your tummy and one on your chest. The hand on your chest should stay as still as possible. The hand on your tummy will go up and down as you breathe.

71

2. Breathe out through your nose (don't force it), and let your tummy fall gently as you do so.
3. Breathe in through the nose letting the tummy rise. Try to make the out breath longer than the in breath.
4. Gradually train yourself to breathe between eight and twelve times per minute.

The aim is to breathe slowly, lifting the abdomen. If you breathe deeply you can become light-headed or your heart may bump a little. This shows how it is not only low carbon dioxide levels but also a rapid change in the levels which can cause symptoms. This is nothing to worry about and if you get in a muddle take a rest and start again.

### Am I getting it right?

People are often anxious about this. Your body will tell you whether or not you are getting it right; you will begin to feel calmer, there might be a few gurglings in your tummy or you might feel muscles letting go of tension but remember, it takes time to achieve this, *it does not happen in the first couple of minutes*.

## Using the breathing to cope with panic attacks

If your attitude is, 'I will die, be sick, faint, wet myself, etc. if I don't fight this panic attack', you will encourage more attacks. It will be a trigger for further attacks, the adrenaline levels will shoot up and it will start all over again. You can train yourself to break this vicious circle. If you are going into a situation you know has caused you to panic before, visualize yourself before you go breathing slowly and coping well. Teach yourself to link the words 'slow breathing' to panic. Write them down together over and over again.

### First aid for panic attacks – using a paper bag

*Exercise*

Make an effort to increase your levels of carbon dioxide by cupping your hands around your nose and mouth, holding a paper (never plastic) bag around your nose and mouth and just **breathe normally**. Do not puff and blow into the bag, you will make your symptoms worse. As you get your own carbon dioxide back from the bag you will feel better.

You can use bag rebreathing to prevent symptoms. Some people use bag rebreathing routinely during the day to prevent attacks. To leave the hands free to read, iron or even so that it is not necessary to hold it while you are watching television you can poke two holes in the upper edge of the bag, strengthen around them with sticky tape to prevent tearing and then attach some elastic. This resembles a horse's nose bag. Some people find the masks used for giving oxygen work well, others use the masks used by painters or people working with dust. These can also be used for a convenient frame for a paper bag. Cut out the middles of the mask and stick the bag around the edge with sticky tape. You can buy these masks at pharmacies or at DIY stores.

Cold water also helps some people. You could splash your face with cold water or put something cold like a bag of frozen peas or an ice pack over your nose and cheeks. Some people find this very helpful to slow down the breathing.

As soon as you feel steadier you must eat or drink something sweet. Why this is only a first-aid measure will be seen in the next section.

# 9

# A Healthy Diet

*How do I eat to keep the blood sugar level stable?*

*(Please note, if your doctor has already given you a diet to follow consult him/her before you make any changes in your eating pattern.)*

It is impossible to give a diet plan that will suit everyone. As long as you keep to the principles of the diet the choice is going to be yours. You might be vegetarian, in which case you will need to add lots of nuts and whole grains; you might be macrobiotic (if either of these you could check for B12 deficiency); you might have a good diet but space your meals badly; or you might be a junk food eater about to reform.

## Principles of the diet

Don't go longer than two-and-a-half to three hours without something to eat. Break your fast between meals, eat a snack as late as possible before bed, and at all times avoid foods and substances that are quickly absorbed into the blood stream in order to minimize rapid changes of the level of glucose in the blood.

- *Avoid or cut down to a minimum refined carbohydrates.*
  Sugar, sweets, chocolate, white bread, white flour, cakes, cookies, pastry, alcohol, sweet drinks, junk foods.
- *Eat non-refined carbohydrates.*
  Non-refined carbohydrates (complex): whole grain cereals, wheat, oats, barley, rice, rye, millet. Give up processed breakfast cereals and make your own muesli from whole oats, nuts, seeds (sunflower, pumpkin or sesame are all very nutritious) and a little dried fruit, sultanas, apricots, etc. Make sure your brown bread is whole grain.
- *Eat protein.*
  Again this is going to be trial and error. Some people feel really well and energetic when they eat more protein. It helps to rid

74

the body of excess water. Others find it does not suit them and they concentrate on complex carbohydrate. Overweight people do well on the Weight Watchers' diet. This includes protein in every meal.

*Animal protein*: Meat, fish, poultry, cheese, eggs, milk, yogurt.
*Vegetable protein*: nuts, seeds, peas, beans, lentils and possibly small amounts in all vegetables.

- *Eat large quantities of vegetables.*
These will supply you with essential minerals and vitamins and provide roughage. Some people have become over-anxious about roughage – bran with everything. This is not a good idea; it can irritate the bowel and hinder the absorption of some minerals. Eating vegetables is a better way to get roughage.
- *Eat lots of fresh fruit.*
Apples are said to be particularly good – the pectin acts as a stabilizer. Although fruit contains quite a lot of sugar, it is in a different form (fructose); it does not need insulin for its digestion, therefore it is an ideal food to help slow down the pancreas.
- *Eat some fat.*
People tend to concentrate on low-fat diets and think this will take care of all cholesterol problems. Yes, cut down on animal fat, but remember there are other factors just as important: stress and a diet low in vegetables and fruit can be just as damaging as moderate amounts of butter. Also remember that some foods actually lower cholesterol levels. They include onions, garlic, apples and olive oil. Olive oil is also wonderful for the immune system – the body's defence against disease.

## Suggested diet

As soon as you get up, or in bed; a small glass of unsweetened juice or piece of fruit.

*Breakfast:* More fruit juice and
Either: *Cooked breakfast:* grilled bacon, fish, eggs, baked beans, cold ham, cheese, or any protein dish plus mushroom or tomatoes. Also one slice of wholemeal bread, two crispbreads, rice cakes etc. with butter or margarine.

Or:　　　　*Cold breakfast:* whole-oat porridge sweetened with a few sultanas or muesli made from whole cereals, nuts, seeds (pumpkin, sunflower, etc.) or plain yogurt with fresh fruit and nuts, fruit yogurt, *fromage frais*, cottage cheese, bread and crispbreads as above.

Weak tea with milk if desired or one cup weak coffee.

*Two hours after breakfast:*

Snack: fruit, yogurt, milk, cheese and biscuits, seeds, nuts.

Lunch:　　　Any protein dish, hot or cold: meat, fish, cheese, eggs, chicken, sardines, tuna, pilchards, etc., or any bean, lentil or nut dish.

All to be eaten with *lots of salad or vegetables*, 1 slice of wholemeal bread or 2 crispbreads.

*Two-and-a-half to three hours after lunch:*

Weak tea, milk with crispbread, cheese, pâté or low-sugar jam, or the same as mid-morning.

*Half an hour before dinner:*

Small glass of fruit juice.

Dinner:　　Same as lunch, plus fruit.

Supper:　　Crispbreads, butter, cheese, pâté, etc. Milk drink, weak tea, herb tea.

This might look like a lot of food, but remember there is no need to eat large quantities. Small and often is the rule.

## *Rules*

* Don't skip meals.
* Eat regularly.
* Avoid sugary foods and drinks, and white flour; cut down on

caffeine, cigarettes (if you must smoke make sure you have eaten), and alcohol.
- Always have protein in your breakfast.
- Never eat a starch-only meal (bread, cake, cereal).

## Other suggestions for blood sugar problems

- *Will any supplements help the blood sugar problem?*
Yes. There is an inexpensive supplement in most health food stores called GTF (Glucose Tolerance Factor); it contains chromium.

   Chromium is also helpful for the once-a-month premenstrual syndrome sufferers. They are often also short of vitamin B3, niacin. B6 100 mgms daily in the premenstrual phase and 50 mgms daily for the rest of the month helps the water retention, and clumsiness. Calcium helps the leg cramps. B6 and potassium both help distended abdomens but as these are both stimulants it is better to take them in the morning. Magnesium can also help the constipation. It is also thought to make the pancreas less sensitive to glucose and thereby slow down the production of insulin. A dose of around 300 mgms daily for six weeks can be helpful. Magnesium can stop the food cravings of PMS. Evening primrose oil is also very helpful for PMS but it might be a couple of months before you feel the benefit of this.

- *Food sensitivities and unstable blood sugar levels*
These can cause troubles. Watch out for palpitations, flushing, bloating, restlessness, insomnia, mood changes and a stuffy nose after certain foods.

- *First aid for unstable blood sugar symptoms*
If there is nothing else but a chocolate bar and you are feeling hungry, say, if you are driving on the motorway, choose one with nuts in it and remember to eat a decent snack as soon as possible. A chocolate bar's effect will last only about an hour.

   If you are out and have a panic attack a cup of tea with sugar must be regarded only as an emergency measure.

- *Macrobiotic diet*
If you can cope with this clean, healthy way of eating which relies mainly on rice and vegetables you will find Michio Kushi and John David Mann's book on blood sugar levels, *Diabetes and Hypoglycaemia: A natural approach*, very interesting.

- *Withdrawal from alcohol or drugs and blood sugar levels*
  It is often difficult to separate the symptoms of withdrawal from those of low blood sugar. After all a large part of a hangover is due to hypoglycaemia. It is therefore essential to be extremely vigilant about your diet if you are in withdrawal from alcohol, street drugs, prescribed drugs (tranquillizers, sleeping pills, antidepressants, or hormone replacement therapy). You stand a much better chance of completing withdrawal and of avoiding panic attacks.

- *Don't try to fit in with other people's eating habits*
  If possible explain to those close to you that you need to keep a steady supply of glucose to the brain to help your nervous system. You are important: ignore any 'are you eating again?' looks. *At all times carry snack foods such as nuts, fruit, crispbread with you.* A salty snack can also keep you going if a meal is late.

- *If you are not convinced*
  Even after painstaking counselling some people are reluctant to accept that their eating style is making their symptoms worse. Some even get annoyed and think their dramatic symptoms cannot possibly be helped by diet. My advice is usually to ask them if they will write down what they have eaten and at what time they ate on the day of the panic attack and the preceding day – it never fails; try it!

# 10

## Conquering Chronic Muscle Spasm

Release makes the energy necessary for change.
Sigmund Freud

## *What have tight muscles to do with panic attacks?*

Some people are unwilling to accept that there is any connection at all and are very resistant to the idea that they are going to have to move in order to get better. I hope you will understand by the end of the chapter the havoc it causes in your nervous system when you walk in a tense manner, sit with your shoulders around your ears and even sleep jaw clenched and knees drawn up. Panic attacks can serve as a warning to make you really look at what is going on in your emotional life.

### *What causes chronic muscle tension?*

A continual state of fear whether it is acknowledged or not. The body does not lie. Imagine a cat stretched out in front of the fire, the muscles relaxed and at their full length. Now imagine a strange dog walks in; the cat jumps to its feet and 'concertinas' ready to spring. You must have seen the cartoon cat Tom (of *Tom and Jerry*) in this attitude many times: back arched, head forward and paws all bunched together. The muscles have contracted because he is afraid. Many of us walk around in a similar contracted state. Clients often react with astonishment when I take them to a mirror to view how they are holding their heads and necks. They have no idea their shoulders are around their ears and their heads are pulled back.

### *What effect does this have?*

Tension or spasm in muscles causes them to be in a contracted state where they cannot, even at rest, go back to their original length and shape. The circulation to the muscles is affected and because the lymphatic drainage is also affected, toxins which are left after the muscles have been nourished cannot be swept away and excreted. These form crystals and cause pain, stiffness and

79

sometimes inflammation and swelling. Muscles in this state are rather like a shirt that has been repeatedly washed in soap powder and not been rinsed. Chronic muscular tension produces not only local muscle pain but also pulls joints out of alignment, causing more pain, and has a profound effect on the mind. Anxiety, panic, dissatisfaction with self and depression result.

### Where does this tension come from?

Chronic muscular tensions can be the effect of present stress or reflections of childhood unhappiness such as rejection, deprivation, frustration, suppression of anger. We put our pain down in the joints and muscles. Tension is sometimes called *armouring* because it restricts movement, stops you displaying your feelings and is some protection from the hurts of life. Armour is the outer edge of your neurosis. I have more to say on neurosis, which really means pain, in my book *Coping with Anxiety and Depression*.

### What happens if I keep the armour on?

Apart from the pain, tension can have other physical effects, such as disturbing the digestion or making the immune system less efficient, but, more importantly, armouring prevents you getting back to the real you, the person you were when you came into the world, the one you were before you donned the suit of armour to protect your vulnerability, the one you were before you were taught to bend your thoughts and feelings to either be acceptable, or come up to the expectations of those around you, before you used the psychological ploys of rationalization, denial or projection – before you shed what has been called 'your first nature'. So now you are saddled with your second nature, how do you get back to where you started? Tension becomes so ingrained in the second nature that we don't notice it.

## How can you shake off this second nature?

A nervous breakdown or a personal crisis is often a good opportunity for a chance to go down (this will be mentioned later), to touch the bottom (you can't go any further than that), and to gain a firm foothold on which to start coming up to emotional health – look at your pain, accept it and start rebuilding.

### What is emotional health?

The ability fully to experience feelings without any mechanisms, without overbreathing, without breath holding, without the armour of chronic muscular tensions, without using chemical relief, without using continual activity, without using relationships – no holding back – being real – getting rid of pretend.

### Taking the armour off

Full breathing and the relaxation of chronic muscular tension releases the energy that is locked into maintaining the armouring. Growth is not possible without giving up the armour of tension. Try the following:

- *Surrender to your body*
  What will happen if I let go? Will I lose control? Will I fall? Some people are afraid to relax because this is often when they take a deep breath. If they have been overbreathing this causes a surge of adrenaline and panic. Many people report panic at the time they sit down to watch television.
- *Open your body*
  Until you open your body, until you choose to live, you cannot fully know yourself; self-realization is impossible without knowing the needs of your inner child. These needs are hidden from you and the constant battle to contain the neurosis which has certainly been your way of coping, but it has also made you anxious and dispirited; you can't keep this charade up any longer.
- *Breathe, let the muscles go – give in*
  Shout, cry, scream if necessary (see *The Primal Scream: Primal therapy, the cure for neurosis* by Dr Arthur Janov). Grounded, integrated or whole people are with their bodies, with their real selves (their inner child), their centre is peaceful – they are not crying inside.

## Owning and caring for your body

On a cramped seventeen-hour flight some years ago a video came on to the screen inviting passengers to do ten minutes of simple aeroplane aerobics. This involved stretching arms up, rotating

81

hands and feet and so on. An embarrassed silence took over and I was interested to see how many people were participating – only six (all women) as far as I could see. People are often so unwilling to acknowledge that their bodies have needs.

### Releasing the tension

Health depends not only on taking in energy in the form of food, oxygen, *prana* and stimulation but also the *discharge* of excess energy. It is so common for anxious people and migraine sufferers to come in saying: I feel as though my body is full of electricity/I feel all charged up/I feel as though I am having tiny electric shocks all over my body/I feel as though I'm going to burst – they are not *discharging*. I usually find such people have extremely tense feet and often painful feet, particularly the instep. The arch is raised; they are not *grounding*.

### Grounding

Bringing energy into the legs and feet stops you being 'all in the head', it gives you a good base, it stabilizes. Releasing the feet provides a safety valve for the discharge of pent-up energy and as tension dissipates, fears, anger and hurt can be expressed. It is only when we discharge our overloaded circuits that we can avoid 'burnout', 'blowing a fuse' or 'exploding'.

### Working with the feet

Reflexology (a type of foot massage which is beneficial to the whole body and very relaxing) is wonderful for tense feet but if you cannot afford this there is a great deal you can do yourself:

- *Foot massage*
  It's a great help to do this twice daily with any oil or moisturizer you have. Spend at least five minutes on each foot and finish with gentle stroking towards the knees. To pamper yourself use aromatherapy oils either in a base oil for massage or to really relax massage them first then have a footbath with a few drops of oil. These essential oils are potent medicine and should be treated as such. Inhalation of the sedative oils is very calming because they work on part of the brain called the limbic system. This incidentally is where tranquillizers work. Aromatherapy

books give full instruction on choosing and mixing oils; see
Further Reading. You can also use alternate hot and cold foot-
baths: two minutes in each for ten minutes.

- *Walking barefooted*
Whenever you can, walk barefooted on grass with your big toes
pointing upwards. This brings the tense arch into contact with
the ground. People who get electric shocks when they touch the
fridge or when they are in shops find this very helpful. Walking
on the shore, particularly on ridged sand, is also beneficial.
Walking in the water is even better; it is very soothing for the
nervous system.
- *Releasing leg tension*
Fear keeps energy out of the legs. Many people lock their
knees feeling they will fall over if they don't. Bringing energy
through the legs can feel threatening for some people. It suggests descent, going down into the unknown, the soul perhaps,
or sadness. Physically going down can also induce fear. To
be lowered to the ground is much more threatening than to be
lifted up, as is going down steps, down in a lift, landing in an
aeroplane. This is possibly all connected to the primitive fear
of falling.
  To free the legs lie on the bed and kick vigorously until you
are tired, or lie on your back in the swimming pool and kick as
hard as you can. You can hold the bar behind you if you are a
non-swimmer.

*Bioenergetic exercises:*
These are described in *Bioenergetics* by Dr Alexander Lowen.
This revolutionary therapy that uses the language of the body to
heal the problems of the mind.

*Exercise 1*

a. Stand on one leg with the knee slightly bent; hold on to the
   chair for support. The leg may tremble; this is tension being
   released. Hold this position until the pain gets too much then
   fall forward on to cushions or blanket.
b. Repeat with other leg.
c. Do exercise a second time.

*Exercise 2*

Bend forward with the knees slightly bent and touch the ground with the fingertips. Try to hold the position until your legs have had a good shake. Rest and repeat.

### Tension in the jaw

Forget all you know about keeping your chin up or having a stiff upper lip. This silly British teaching is just a way of stopping you crying – what's wrong with crying? If pollen gets up your nose you sneeze – pain hurts, why not cry?

A tense jaw won't allow this. You need to drop your chin before you can give in to some good therapeutic sobs. Think of how a baby's lower lip quivers and drops just before it cries. People with compressed lips are said to be tight-lipped. This can serve to hold in what you really want to say, also as a guard against 'swallowing' what other people are saying. A set jaw is thought to be a sign of strength – people 'take it on the jaw'. A tight jaw can be very uncomfortable. To relax it pretend to yawn; this makes air rush into the lungs and also helps to release the tension. To prevent your jaw tightening up again place tongue just behind front teeth.

### Crying

Are you only able to cry when you are really pushed hard and then are you angry with the person, possibly even yourself, who pushed you? Does it feel like failure? Does it feel like weakness?

You might say no, that is not like me, I am always crying. But what about the quality of that crying? Is it just the overflow you are discharging? There will be no real release until the energy that is crushing your feelings comes away in sobs that rock your being, sobs that come from way down in your solar plexus, noisy and uncontrolled.

Until you can commit yourself to working with your body to open the cage and release the imprisoned emotions you cannot expect to be either physically or psychologically well.

### Tension in the scalp

Hold your head with fingers meeting at the midline. Move scalp from side to side. Massage temples, brow, behind ears and the base of the skull, then go all over head as though you were washing your hair. Open eyes wide in an expression of fear; and then relax.

### Tension in the shoulders

When the shoulders and brow are raised and the head is pushed forward, this is an attitude of fear. Around the base of the skull where the head and neck join the muscles become very sore. The headaches and symptoms due to lack of circulation to the brain have been discussed earlier.

Where the neck joins the shoulders the tightening of the anterior, middle and posterior scalene muscles has the effect of a rope around the neck. The tightening of these muscles cramps the upper ribs and affects the breathing by constricting the opening to the chest. It can also affect the voice.

*To release the shoulders:*

a. Breathe in slowly, raising the shoulders; let them drop as you breathe out.
b. Hang arms limply by your sides, imagine there is a piece of chalk on the tip of your shoulders, draw clockwise circles.
c. Stand up and do 'windmills' with your arms.

If you can get to a pool it is good to do these exercises in water.

### Head, neck and shoulder massage

If you can find a friend to give you the simple massage that follows you will find great benefit. Some people don't attempt massage because they feel only trained people can do it. This is not so, anyone can bring relief to tight muscles. There are, however, a few don'ts.

*Don'ts*
• Don't massage over broken skin, varicose veins, where there is inflammation, over the heart, over the tummy, on the front of the neck, if there is malignant disease.
• Don't get tense as you work – breathe slowly and relax – you will be much more effective.

- Remember you are bringing the blood to the tight muscles – bringing fresh water to rinse the shirt full of soap crystals.

## Instructions for the helper

When you have done this massage a few times you will be able to feel the tense muscles; they feel gluey or harder and resist the pressure of your fingers. Just work away in these areas and you will feel the muscles becoming less taut. Your fingers are bringing more blood to the area and allowing waste products to be taken away.

Don't be concerned about technique. If your thoughts are gentle towards your partner and you desire to help him/her you cannot do any harm; just follow the above rules and let your fingers take over.

Be as relaxed as you can; let your breath out as you drop your shoulders; balance your partner's head, make sure her back is straight but slack, press her shoulders gently down.

1. Take the energy down to the feet by massaging under the instep in a circular motion and then give both feet a brisk rub. If the person can't bear her feet massaged just hold with the backs of your hands together so that your fingers press into the instep.

2. Stand behind your partner, hold the head in both hands with the fingers meeting at the top and move the scalp from side to side. Then move your fingers all over the scalp as if you were washing her hair.

3. Support her forehead with your left hand if you are right-handed. Use the opposite hand if you are left-handed. Ask your partner to 'give' you her head – to drop her head on to your hand.

4. With thumb and index finger press firmly (as shown) on the bone at the base of the skull. Hold these points for about fifteen seconds then stretch hand to reach the bone behind the ears. Hold again, then press thumb into the 'salt cellar' at the top of the spine where the head joins the neck. Massage in a circular motion. Continue to support the forehead; massage

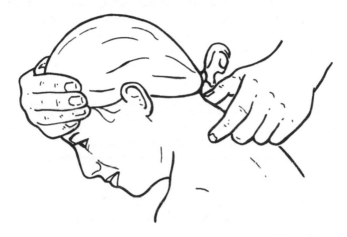

quite firmly at the base of the skull using the thumb and fingers; make small circular movements.

5. Now move on to the back of the neck using the thumb and index finger on either side of the neck bones; hold for about fifteen seconds, then hold where the neck joins the shoulders. Then go over neck again using a circular movement.

6. Place your hands over the shoulders with the fingers pointing towards the chest and use the thumb or heel of the hand to knead the muscles in a circular motion. I call this the motion picture bit. You must have seen many screen idols having their shoulders massaged like this.

   Get feedback from your partner; see if she would like you to go back to any sore place.

7. Put one arm across the top of your partner's chest and encourage them to relax forward on to it. With the other hand continue massaging down the side of (but not on) the bones of the spine. Work in a similar fashion around the shoulder blade. Use the other arm and repeat for the other side of the spine.

8. Stand in front of your partner, pick up the wrist and shake the hand letting it flop (unless there is pain in the joint) and

ask them to imagine a wet sweater on the washing line. You will feel the arm become heavier when they think 'heavy'. Stretch the palm area, give the fingers a gentle pull and then massage the hand. Next hold the hand and with your other hand hook your thumb into the armpit. Give the arm a gentle pull. Repeat for the other side.

9. Stand behind your partner. Support her head against your chest. Massage the temples in a circular fashion, then stroke the brow with both first fingers from the centre outwards. To release tension in the jaw stroke or massage from the chin to behind the ear.

10. Finish off with magnetic massage by stroking lightly and rapidly from the head down the back and then down the arms and hands.

Sometimes people are quite sleepy after a head and neck massage. Your partner might need a short rest before helping you.

For the very tense person, it is a great help to have a massage daily. The therapeutic value of massage is becoming more recognized in this country. Aromatherapy, massaging with the essential oil of plants, has been proved to have a beneficial effect on the nervous system (see the exercise on page 108).

### Further exercises

• *Quick tension release*
  This can be done anywhere – on a bus, in a meeting. Sit down with your back straight but not stiff, put your hands palm upwards in your lap and place your feet together flat on the floor. Droop your head a little, take a slow complete breath and as you let it out let your shoulders drop and allow your thighs and knees to fall outwards. Imagine a beautiful, blue sparkling light which starts about a foot (30 cm) above your head; let it ripple through your body and out of the soles of your feet into the floor and it will take your tension with it. If you practise this regularly you will be surprised how effective it is. You may also notice it makes your feet tingle. Alternatively, you could do the wet dog shake.

88

- *The wet dog shake*
  Imagine you are an Old English sheepdog (a Dulux dog); you have been in the sea and now you are shaking the water out of your coat. Picture the dog – he shakes from head to tail. You do the same; hold on to something if you need to, then change hands. Really let go and feel your cheeks wobble. If you are a back sufferer take it gently.
- *Laughter*
  Laughter is a great muscle relaxant. It also gives all your internal organs a massage.

## Tight muscles pull bones out of alignment

The skeletal system provides a movable framework which gives support and protection to the soft tissues. The spine, which consists of thirty-three irregular bones, serves as the main support for the trunk and neck, and gives protection to the spinal cord.

### The backbone

Although each joint allows only a slight movement because there are so many of them it is flexible and allows the trunk to move freely – at least this is how it should be. So many people are afraid to move their spines and suffer back pain and sciatica as a result.

### The backbone's connected to the ...

Everything. The spinal nerves leave the spinal cord in pairs to service the whole body: the neck and arms from the neck or cervical area; the abdomen and rib-cage from the thoracic or chest area; the lower back, hips and legs from the lumbar area, and the back of the legs from the sacral area. This should give you some idea of the area of the spine your symptoms may be coming from; a pain in the knee for example might have nothing to do with the knee but be coming from the spine and a pain in the head or face can have its origins in the neck.

### How can this cause panic attacks?

Osteopaths and chiropractors believe that a straight, flexible spine means a healthy body and that slight displacements of vertebrae, called subluxations, interfere with the nerve supply and can cause organic disease. Sometimes local pain in the spine is not a feature and malfunctions of the internal organs are the first sign. The symptoms caused by these displacements correspond to the vertebrae concerned; for example, displacements of the atlas, the first bone of the spine, can impede the flow of blood in the cerebral arteries and cause migraine. The commonest cause of this displacement is repeatedly turning the head to one side to look at a badly placed television set or notes at the side of a computer. Lying on the tummy in bed and keeping the head in one position is another cause. Because the circulation to the head is affected it can also cause dizziness, and we have seen how becoming dizzy when you are outside is a potent trigger for a panic attack. If you have stiffness or pain in the neck and dizziness when you turn your head see your doctor first and if he/she cannot help you, have your neck adjusted by an osteopath or chiropractor. Your doctor may be able to recommend one.

*Summary*

There is no short cut to unlocking muscles and finding emotional health. Many have tried drugs for this purpose but, as has been said, the outcome is a compounding of the muscle spasm *and* the emotional problems. It is scary to let go and many times you will want to retreat to your prison and firmly lock the gates – don't – come out and try again. Don't be put off by people who feel threatened by the change in you; your first duty is to your inner child. There will be others who will welcome the new you.

# 11

## Agoraphobia

### What is agoraphobia?

Agoraphobia literally means fear of the assembly or market place, but the term is generally used to describe extreme fear of leaving the safety of the home. It can be a manifestation of severe anxiety or depression, or can appear in a person who feels quite well until they try to venture outdoors. Such people are often quite happy to go out if there is someone with them. Agoraphobia is an extremely distressing problem; the sufferer loses freedom, self-reliance, self-esteem and also suffers physically through lack of light, fresh air, exercise and sunshine.

### Should I see the doctor?

Yes. He/she will be able to tell you whether you are suffering from anxiety or depression, or both, and might feel you need help from drugs for a while just to get you back into a more normal routine. The dangers of long-term drug treatment have already been discussed.

Your doctor might also refer you to a psychologist or nurse-therapist who could support you with counselling or desensitization therapy. This treatment is relaxation training plus gradual exposure to the situations you fear most, such as going into a shop or travelling on a bus. You would be asked to make a list of everything you have to face which makes you afraid. Starting with the least fearsome, together you would gradually work through the list.

If your doctor cannot help you and you have already tried drugs you have nothing to lose and perhaps a great deal to gain if you use the following suggestions. **Remember many people come through agoraphobia with nothing more than self-help**. Before you can progress you need to accept the fact that although you might not even remember the incident there is a memory tucked away in some corner of your mind which makes you react with fear in certain situations. If you are terribly anxious about everything and going out just happens to be included you will need professional help, but that does not mean that you would not benefit from using self-help methods too. In the same way that a tune or smell can bring back a memory you thought you had forgotten, the *thought* of being in a certain place or doing something, such as travelling on the Underground, can dredge up a fear despite the fact that you might have no clear memory of when it originated.

## What plants these rogue thoughts in the mind?

When agoraphobia is not part of a generally very anxious state people can often remember the first time they had funny feelings outside. One man said he remembered the identical feeling many years ago when he played in the street soon after he had measles. He was six years old at the time. Another man said he first had the feelings when he was twelve when on a Sunday School outing he had been hit by a cricket bat. The feeling came again when as an adult he witnessed a car crash. It is often when people are physically low that they have their first panic attacks outside; after 'flu is very common.

### When thoughts work in your favour

If you are at home and you decide to play tennis or go out dancing try just *thinking* about what you are going to do, for example: My new tennis shoes are upstairs, I'll give Bill a ring ...; or, Julie might be at the dance, it was fun last time ...; and so on. This releases the chemicals in your brain necessary for you to run for the ball, rock the night away, or whatever. Think of it: even before your bottom leaves the chair this is happening; it's an exciting thought because it should explain what happens in agoraphobia.

### When your thoughts work against you

Again imagine you are sitting at home and you think with dread: I have to go to the meeting/supermarket/to post a letter/to the corner shop/to get my pension/to that party/to London/I hate going out/ I'll never cope/I might be sick/I might faint ... What do you think the body is being flooded with in response to these thoughts? Yes, adrenaline. So the fear these thoughts bring triggers overbreathing and then the pulse races, you sweat and all the dreaded feelings invade your mind. Think of it: this is before you even leave your chair – there is no real threat at all. In his article 'Hyperventilation Syndromes in Medicine and Psychiatry' (see page 39) Professor Lum states that 60% of agoraphobes hyperventilate and 60% of hyperventilators are agoraphobic.

This includes Jill!

> ### Dear Agony Aunt – I'm An Agoraphobe
>
> It's panic that's driving me crazy,
> I haven't been out for a week!
> At the thought of crossing the threshold
> My breathing speeds up and I freak!

I know agoraphobia is extremely distressing and frustrating and you can be as much a prisoner with this as you would be with two broken ankles, but consider it: changing your thinking would not get rid of the fratures, but **changing your thoughts could stop you overbreathing, stop you panicking and *cure* your agoraphobia**. Let's stop using this term and talk about panicky feelings at the thought of going out, because that is *all* they are. Some people talk about 'my agoraphobia' and feel affronted when I demystify it. They would rather think of it as an illness in itself rather than a symptom of overstimulated nerves   something that needs effort to improve. Fortunately most people are delighted to have all anxiety symptoms explained and love the feeling that they can be in control.

## How can I change my thoughts?

I don't pretend this is easy but it can be done. It involves accepting what was said about the brain releasing helpful chemicals when you give it the right thoughts, relaxation, visualization, and lots and lots of practice.

### Relaxation and visualization

Visualization means making mental pictures to lead your body in the direction in which you want it to go; for example if you are low in energy, during relaxation when your body is ready to respond you would visualize yourself active and fit, absorbed in your favourite sport, dancing or running, and so on. If you wanted to quieten an overactive nervous system you could imagine you were drifting on a calm lake, floating wrapped in a fluffy pink cloud, or that you were a baby being gently rocked in a crib. If you had a fever you could imagine a cool mountain stream was washing over you, or if you had a pain you could imagine you were breathing soft pink light into the sore place and then you were sending it out through the soles of your feet into the ground on the outbreath. Don't dismiss these suggestions as fanciful – visualization can be very powerful. Choosing the right images is as personal as choosing the right diet; you know your fears, you know what will make you feel safe.

### How can I practise this at home?

1. When you are not hungry and when you do not need the lavatory, find a warm quiet place, either lying or sitting. Cover yourself with a blanket or extra sweater.
2. Choose your image – your safe place. If you don't like any of the previous suggestions, what about lying on warm sand surrounded by a windbreak listening to the sea, or in a walled garden listening to summer sounds? When you are where you want to be practise gentle complete breaths for ten minutes.
3. When you feel warm and relaxed imagine yourself going into the situation you fear and start self-talk. Continuing to breathe slowly repeat whatever you need to say several times – statements such as: I am calm/this is easy/Mary, you are doing so well/better and better every day in every way/and so on; any words of comfort, praise and reassurance you feel you would like to hear, until the old fear is erased and new confident, calm thoughts gleam like jewels in your mind. If there are many situations which make you panic start with the one which is the least fear provoking and as you conquer one, move on to the next.
4. Practise day after day. **Don't give up after two days and say this is not working – it takes *time*.**

You might think this is not a very long chapter to cover such an enormous problem. Agoraphobia is a panic attack outside or at the thought of going outside – aspects of panic attacks have been covered in other chapters: breathing, unstable blood sugar levels, and tight muscles. If you are looking after these you should be more than half way to curing your agoraphobia.

For more on this topic, read *Overcoming Agoraphobia* by Melissa Murphy (Sheldon Press).

# 12
## Worry, Worry, Worry

In headaches and worry life leaks away.
W. H. Auden

Worry is a reaction to a problem that we don't have an answer to. In an attempt to find a solution the brain works overtime and the thought process is speeded up. This goes without saying; it would be hard to imagine anyone worrying slowly.

### Background worry and panic

It is easy to see why the constant worrier is more likely to have panic attacks. He/she is already half-way there. It is only one small step from negative thoughts such as 'life's always hard', 'I'm useless', to 'I can't cope', 'I'm going to faint.'

We have talked a lot about the biological approach to panic, the effect of breathing, the blood sugar, the muscles, nutrition and supplements. It is time now to discuss how you can promote yourself to managing director; how you can retrain your fearful thoughts and order them to give up old habits and work with you instead of against you.

### Worry: productive and unproductive

A degree of productive worry is good if it is really only used for problem solving. For example, imagine you are in the middle of a busy day at work when a glance at your diary reminds you of a dinner party you had arranged for that evening. You barely know the couple but had enjoyed meeting them so much that you wanted to get better acquainted. Your mind starts to spin when you realize the house is like Paddy's market, there's a tub of margarine and half of last night's pizza in the fridge, a lot of ice cubes but nothing else in the freezer, your hair needs washing and your only decent dress is at the cleaner's. Do you get the feeling? Because you are worried, the problem solving starts: The house, what a mess; I could ring Lucy and ask her to do a quick tidy-up for me. Oh dear, the meal, I'll never do it in time; I could raid Marks and Spencer's at lunchtime – but – no home cooking, I can't do that: I could if I dressed it up a bit, no one would know – spot of cream and a few chives in the soup and ... and if I ring them now and ask them if they can make it eight o'clock instead of seven-thirty (but what will they think if I do that?), I can collect my dress on the way home and if I wash my hair as soon as I get in it should be fine by eight – worry, worry, worry – all done – problem solved.

The opposite of this is unproductive worry. This can start as looking for a solution and then get out of hand. What if there is no solution to the problem, or there is not necessity for action, and yet the worry drones on and on, around and around, like a hamster on a wheel? This is the type of worry we need to get rid of. The trouble is, the thought process is often so ingrained that we become almost addicted to it – it is what we *know*, and at the slightest anxiety or even without an apparent trigger we worry, worry, worry. The thoughts of the constant worrier are often:

- What if she dies before me?
- What if I miss that train?
- What if the dog gets run over?
- If I say no I'll hurt her feelings.
- What will Mrs Jones think?
- I haven't the confidence to do that.
- I must hide my feelings.
- Life is so embarrassing.
- I feel such pain and fear when I see the pain of others.
- I keep imagining all these horrible things happening.
- I can never look on the bright side.
- What if I fail?
- What if I have a panic attack?
- What if something awful happens?
- What if there's an earthquake?
- What if I wear that suit and it gets a mark on it?

### A million 'what ifs'

Worrying like this is called anticipatory anxiety. This type of anxiety is understandable if you are afraid of the dentist and your appointment is coming uncomfortably close, but the majority of things people worry about in this way are the result of fearful, negative thoughts which in turn are the result of an exhausted nervous system. It would be impossible for someone whose nervous system was in a healthy state to spend the day worrying about a succession of events that it is extremely unlikely will come to pass; they would be relaxed and just getting on with life, possibly even thinking about how pleasurable or productive they could make their day.

## The way forward

You are probably only too aware that entreaties to stop worrying or bullying, 'for goodness sake stop worrying – you worry about every little thing', make you feel a great deal worse because they add guilt and blame to a way of being that is very unhappy, a state you would very much like to change if you knew how. It's like asking someone not to cough when they have bronchitis!

### Acceptance

The first step is to accept that excessive worry is a symptom not an inevitable part of being you; when your nerves recover you will worry less. If you have no counsellor or person who can keep gently reminding you of this, then write notes to yourself and put them on the fridge door, by the telephone and on your bedside table. Acceptance is vital: you cannot take the next step without fully believing that worrying about the worrying and continually looking inward for solutions, going over and over the symptoms, will just compound your problem. Fear → adrenaline → more fear. Relaxation → peace → more relaxation. In a panic attack you have experienced the worst of the symptoms of anxiety; there is a limit to how many awful feelings there are, although you might find it hard to believe that. How could acceptance of worrying or panic make it any worse? Think about what you have read about how your body reacts to your mood.

Millions of nervous sufferers have found Dr Claire Weekes' book *Self Help for Your Nerves* (see Further Reading) a great comfort and many have regained their health with the help of this alone. She stressed the need to go along with the feelings and not fight them. Fighting them tenses up the muscles, speeds up the breathing and so on – all the damaging triggers that by now you should know so well. These feelings will not kill you, they will not make you ill; allow them to happen and repeat something like, 'It will pass, it will pass'. Only when you give up fighting will they lessen in intensity, and finally you will be in control.

Claire Weekes' formula was:  **ACCEPTANCE**
**FLOATING**
**LETTING TIME PASS**.

### Floating

Some people say, 'But how do you "float"?' It is really what it says, floating along with the feelings, moving with them and coming out the other side. You will see that far from losing control, you *gain* control – I'm not afraid of you; you are only feelings; you will vanish when I learn to relax more and stop worrying. This takes practice and courage, and remember you are the only one who can slow your breathing, you are the only one who can let tight muscles go. Choose an image to help you float, perhaps see yourself in a boat floating down a gently flowing river; or safe in a pink fluffy cloud; or holding the hand of a trusted friend. Visualize yourself in your floating scene several times a day and link it to a short command, for example 'boat'. This in time will replace the panicky thoughts: I can't cope, I'll be sick, and so on. The negative images and thoughts need to be firmly and repeatedly replaced by comforting thoughts and relaxing images.

Worrying is like any other nervous habit; just as the nail biter's fingers keep straying unbidden to his/her mouth, so the worrying thoughts come uninvited into the mind and start their endless chatter. When you 'wake up' (bring them into your conscious mind) and discuss these thoughts with yourself, you can order them to 'stop' or 'go away'.

### Letting time pass

This is very difficult for the nervous person. Yes, you are desperate to get rid of these awful feelings, but unfortunately it takes time; you will have to be patient. You will also have to accept that there will be times when you think it's not going to work and you feel as far back as ever. Nature does not heal in straight lines

– it's normal to go up and down. Keep in mind the physiological fact nervous tissue takes longer to heal than skin, muscles or bones. This might help you to keep things in perspective.

### Can the people around help?

Yes. Ask them gently to remind you to relax when the worrying thoughts start to spill out. You might feel slightly irritated or hurt when they do this but it will serve to help your awareness of the problem and it will also prevent what commonly happens in this situation, namely that the sufferer goes on and on, the onlooker keeps quiet until he/she can stand it no longer and then explodes. This is disastrous for all concerned. Gentle reminders that talking about the symptoms all the time just reinforces them are more helpful. Bear in mind that in continually talking about the symptoms the sufferer is looking for a way out, an answer, and he/she might think you unfeeling if you take this approach. The sufferer will learn more by having constant reassurance withdrawn. Suggest a time that the feelings can be discussed. Keep to that time although it might produce anger or tears. The important message for the sufferer is, 'The answer is within you'. The most positive thing the carer can do is to read the book and work with the sufferer; do the exercises and listen to relaxation CDs together.

# 13
## Exercise, Daylight, Sunlight, Fresh Air

### *Exercise*

When people realize they are inviting the disease process to take over if they don't exercise they become much more committed to it. When you slow down your circulation by inactivity, organic function, the digestion, for example, becomes sluggish; this causes constipation. Muscles are also affected, not only by lack of nourishment, but also by a build-up of crystals which are formed from the waste products of digestion. The rubbish disposal system of the body is called the lymphatic system.

### Why does the lymphatic system need movement?

The lymphatic system is part of the body's defence against disease. A body fluid called lymph, which relies on muscle contraction for its circulation, is carried through a complex network of small vessels which carry cellular refuse on the way. It is then passed into the bloodstream where it is processed. Unlike the circulatory system, the lymphatic system has no pump; if you don't move then the lymph slows down. The results can be a collection of fluid in the tissues, particularly around the ankles if you have been sitting, a depressed immune system, and some cells in the body which rely on lymph for their nourishment become malnourished. Even if you have to stay in bed for some reason you can still help to circulate the lymph by gently squeezing each group of muscles in turn, and rotating the ankles and wrists. Massage can also be very helpful.

### Start slowly

Take care not to rush into frenetic activity if you have been sitting around for months. Some conditions, for instance ME, do not respond to exercise, but, in saying that, there are few problems which do not respond to gentle exercise. Check with your doctor if you are unsure. Build up the amount of exercise slowly. Some people are so out of touch with their bodies that they are very resistant to the idea of exercise.

101

*Gentle movements sitting down with visualization*

If you have been inactive perhaps you could start with exercises sitting down. As you do this routine, visualize anything that suggests improved circulation; slow streams becoming fast flowing sparkling rivers, pipes being unblocked, or anything that comes to mind. Bring life to your circulation.

*Exercise*

1. Place your feet in front of you about a foot (30 cm) apart. Drop your shoulders and look at the floor a few feet (1 m) in front of you; this stops you shortening the muscles at the side of the neck – part of the iron collar of tension.

2. Take one complete breath (breathing in through the nose, imagine the breath rising up through the feet, lift out abdomen, then ribs and then take breath up into shoulders), open your mouth as you let the breath out and imagine you are filled with the bright colour of your choice.

3. Breathe normally, lift the shoulders towards the ears and let them drop towards the floor; eight times if you can.

4. Keeping the arm limp, circle each shoulder in a clockwise direction eight times, and then try doing them together.

5. To stretch the neck allow your head to fall to the right, bring it back to the centre, then allow it to drop to the left; four times each side. Don't raise your shoulder to meet your ear.

6. Stretch both arms to the ceiling and let them fall loosely towards the floor.

7. Stretch out the fingers, then draw eight circles, both ways, with the forefingers.

8. To exercise the legs, draw the same circles with each big toe in turn.

9. For the buttocks and thighs tighten these muscles and feel yourself rise in your seat.

10. Finish by shaking all over like a wet dog.

Fear of shaking in public is often the reason for people staying indoors. Regularly doing the wet dog exercise is very helpful. It takes a lot more energy to hold shaking in than to let it out. Have a good shake whenever you feel tense and particularly before any social event you are worried about. If you are in trouble when you are out find a lavatory where you can let your jaw go loose and allow yourself to shake from the head down.

If you don't want to make special time to exercise you could start building exercise into your daily life, a few stretches, shakes or wrist and foot movements at your desk, when watching television, at the kitchen sink, while you are on the telephone or waiting for the kettle to boil. These exercises are useful if you do not feel up to swimming, walking or more strenuous exercise. Remember what happens to your circulation if you don't move. Perhaps the next stage could be walking briskly for thirty minutes daily and then progressing to aerobic exercise. It is easier and safer to have some supervision. Join a class or take the advice of the fitness coach at a leisure centre. The exercises might feel like a terrible chore at first, but just keep going; when you feel the benefits you will be more enthusiastic.

## Daylight

Biologists have discovered that light is not only essential to our health but also that individual requirements for light vary as much as individual requirements for vitamins. Daylight is necessary for the normal functioning of the brain and for the regulation of the wake–sleep cycle; it therefore compounds your nervous problems if you are housebound with agoraphobia. Even if you are severely agoraphobic you can sit at an open window, without your spectacles, for at least twenty minutes in the brightest part of the day. Also avoid turning day into night. This gives you a feeling of being permanently jet-lagged and depressed. It's hard to get out of bed in the morning if you are depressed, but it is the only way to progress (see my *Coping with Anxiety and Depression*).

## Sunlight

Sunlight lifts the mood, makes vitamins, kills germs and revitalizes us.

It is foolish to lie and bake in the sun for long periods, but unless you have a sun allergy it is unwise to walk around covered in sun block, wearing dark glasses.

## Fresh air

Much has been said about breathing. When you are taking your wonderful complete breaths don't do it where there is stale air. Air contaminated by smoke or fumes is easily recognized, but there are other causes of stale air which are not so well known.

### Positive ions

Air contains positively and negatively charged particles. We breathe in these particles and absorb them through our skin (interestingly enough at acupuncture points). If there is an excess of positively charged particles, as there is before a storm, during spells of hot wind, in 'sick' buildings where computers and other electrical equipment are in badly ventilated rooms, the positively charged particles dominate. This causes not only respiratory problems but also headaches, irritability, digestive problems, anxiety and depression. The effect on the nervous system is powerful and is why this can be a trigger for panic attacks.

The brain overproduces a chemical called serotonin and this can produce nasal congestion, lethargy, feeling sticky (not the same feeling as being too hot) and swollen. The oppressive feeling before an electrical storm best describes this – a restless feeling, being 'under the weather'. We can also experience this in cities where stale air is trapped between tall buildings, or sitting in badly stuffy rooms surrounded by plastic and electrical equipment, wearing clothes made from synthetic fibres.

### Negative ions

Negative ions have a tonic effect on the nervous system and reduce histamine levels in the blood. As any allergy sufferer knows, histamine is strongly associated with unpleasant feelings.

The benefits of negative ionization are becoming widely known, not only for cleaning the air, killing bacteria and viruses, but also as a treatment for asthma, bronchitis, migraine, burns, scalds and wounds. Sufferers from Irritable Bowel Syndrome could also benefit from negatively charged air. An interesting book on this subject called *The Ion Effect* by Fred Soyka describes the effect of positive ions on the mind and body.

### *Weather-sensitive people*

After a thunderstorm the air is negatively charged; it smells fresh and we experience 'the calm after the storm', our energy returns and our mood improves. The air by the sea, waterfalls and flowing water, even the shower, is also negatively charged and can produce a feeling of well-being. Some people are more affected by this than others, in the same way that some people are irritable and restless when the moon is full and others do not notice it. At full moon the positively charged layer of the ionosphere, air and particles which absorb harmful radiation from the sun, is pushed nearer the earth, thus increasing the number of positive ions in the air we breathe.

### *Avoid being bombarded with positive ions*

Keep your home well ventilated and avoid nylon sheets, carpets and clothes if possible. At work, take frequent breaks from computer screens, fit a screen filter and buy an ionizer (a small machine that negatively charges the air). Ionizers are available in most large stores; you may have to look in a health magazine or office suppliers for an address for a filter. If you drive a lot you could fit a small ionizer in the car. This greatly reduces the effects of pollution and car sickness. Many drivers have reported that they feel less tired at the end of the day.

You cannot overdo negative ions. There is no maximum dosage, you can breathe in as many as you like. Some people have ionizers in every room. If you have one in your sitting room don't forget to put it by your bed at night; they do help you to have a restful night.

### *What else can I do to get rid of positive ions?*

Walking by the sea and taking a shower have been mentioned

earlier. You could also try what is known as magnetic massage. This simply means stroking with the finger tips using a feather-light touch from the top of the head down the arms, chest and abdomen as far as you can reach and flicking your hands after a few strokes to throw off the positive ions. If you don't do this they will become heavy and sticky. Do this for anyone who is restless or has a headache and it will be greatly appreciated. There is a limit to how much you can reach when you are doing it for yourself but for someone else it is useful to stroke from the head to the base of the spine; take your hands to the side then shake away what you have collected. Do this for about five minutes then wash your hands. Invariably the recipient says they feel lighter after this massage. If after using this you become interested in using your hands you could ask the library to order you a copy of Dolores Krieger's book *The Therapeutic Touch: How to use your hands to help or to heal*. It is rather wordy, but don't be put off by that because it does give information about using the human energy field for healing. This is a fascinating subject. Bookshops can also order this book. Dolores Krieger is professor emerita of nursing at New York University; she first researched this subject in the seventies and gave it the name 'therapeutic touch'.

## Therapeutic touch

Our hearts, brains, muscles and nerves all run on a delicate form of electricity, so it follows that whilst we do not need to be plugged into a socket in the wall to operate we are still electrical beings and are surrounded by an electromagnetic field. In the 1930s a Russian called Kirlian experimented with photography which clearly showed this field. One of the first people to study what he called the L-fields or the fields of life, and how they affect health, was Harold Saxon Burr of Yale University Medical School. Dr Robert O. Becker, a leading modern researcher on electromagnetic pollution, believes that man-made electromagnetic fields from power lines and electrical appliances can cause depression, a depressed immune system and other health problems. The research of this man and others suggests that disturbances in the electrical field develop before illness in the physical body. This could be the medicine of the future, the prevention and treatment of illness through correcting faults in the electromagnetic field. This knowledge is not new, and similarities can be found in ancient forms of healing.

### Can I feel my own electrical field?

Only 1% of people can't, so try it. You might have to try on a few occasions before you can be sure, but the more you practise, the more sensitive your hands will become. The movement used to build up the field between the hands is as if you were playing a concertina slowly:

*Exercise*

1. Sit in an upright chair with your back straight but not tense, drop your shoulders and breathe slowly from the abdomen. If you can continue to do this whilst you are following the rest of the exercise it would be better, but if you can't fit it in with the rest just do a few slow breaths before you start.

2. Stretch your fingers out wide and become aware of the palms of your hands.

3. Rub your hands together briskly for about fifteen seconds.

4. Hold the hands about eight inches (20 cm) apart then gradually bring them towards each other until they are about one inch (2.5 cm) apart, but do not let them touch.

5. Separate the hands again, this time to about six inches (15 cm) apart and then bring them towards each other, again without touching.

6. This time bring them together again and bounce them together; remember to keep the hands relaxed. You will feel a resistance or a feeling of pressure between your hands. Some people say they feel as if there is foam rubber between their hands, others describe feelings of heat, tingling, throbbing or pulling.

### Using therapeutic touch on yourself

This is very like the magnetic massage, the same flowing movements, but this time you don't touch the body. Now that your hands are energized you can use them to clear congestion, increase

107

relaxation, and ease discomfort. Take a few complete breaths and consciously think about caring for yourself.

*Exercise*

1. Have a footbath with five drops of lavender or marjoram essential oil, or simply massage under the arch for about a minute. If your feet are very tense take a little longer over it then place them flat on the floor if sitting.

2. Sit relaxed or lie on the floor or bed; slow down your breathing.

3. Close your eyes and imagine yourself totally well and peaceful. If you cannot get this image, give yourself the command: I am totally well and peaceful; and imagine a pure white light is entering your head, filling your body and coming from your fingers and palms. Reach up beyond your head and stroke about three to four inches above your body just as though you were touching it; down over your face, neck, chest and abdomen, and then sweep the hands to either side of the body; this is important because you need to take the congestion clear of your body. You will feel prickling or heat in your hands as you pick up congestion. You can just flick this off as though you are shaking water from your hands, in the same way you did for magnetic massage.

4. Continue stroking for about ten minutes or until your arms feel tired.

5. Now, still imagining you are filled with white light, place your hands at the top of your thighs where they join the body and if you can cross your left foot over your right comfortably, do. If not, then just have the feet touching. Stay there for as long as you feel you want to.

There is a great deal of research going on at the moment on therapeutic touch. It is a gentle, non-drug, inexpensive treatment which not only has a profound effect on the nervous system but is also soul therapy for so many people. If you deny you have a soul or spirit and think you only have a body and personality, then the next chapter is not for you.

# 14

## Loving the Inner Child

> The truth about our childhood is stored up in our body and although we can repress it, we can never alter it. Our intellect can be deceived, our feelings manipulated ... But some day the body will present its bill, for it is as incorruptible as a child who, still whole in spirit, will accept no compromise or excuses, and it will not stop tormenting us until we stop evading the truth.
>
> Margaret Atwood, *True Stories*

### *Who are you?*

We have seen that when we let go of the protection of rigid muscles and shallow breathing we can feel enormous emotional release and be much nearer to finding out who we really are. Another way we can get nearer to our real being is to make a conscious, loving decision to get to know the spirit of the child in us who was 'squashed'; to connect again with the spontaneity and joy which is the birthright of every human being. Growth is not possible without pain, it is scary and difficult to leave behind the outgrown thoughts that have kept us cemented behind our wall of neuroses. Part of the fear is that if we open up and go down to soul level we don't know how much is going to be there; it's 'like springing the lock on Pandora's box' – will it overwhelm us, will it kill us, what will be there, will it be worse than where we are now? All these questions make us want to keep the protection up, to settle down again behind the wall, *but at what cost*: physical illness, chronic anxiety, depression, disintegration of the personality?

You could choose to half-live, but to be whole something has to give. I don't pretend it is easy to clear away years of accumulated soul garbage, the garbage we have kept there by all our physical mechanisms, our addictions, not just to drink, drugs and food, but also to work, relationships, perfection, exercise, compulsive talking. Our lack of inner vision also keeps us firmly stuck where we are.

## How can I make contact with the child within?

A helpful book on this is *Healing Your Aloneness: Finding love and wholeness through your inner child* by Erica J. Chopich and Margaret Paul. It helps you to build a nurturing balance between the adult in you and your inner child. It describes a self-healing process which can be used every day to get rid of self-destructive patterns and take away fears.

Another valuable book is Louise Hay's *You Can Heal Your Life*. She teaches that we are 100% responsible for all our experiences and that every thought we think is creating our future. She says that the point of power is in the present moment and that when we really love ourselves, everything in our life works. She also stresses that we must release the past and forgive everyone.

Some people have been able to bring together the adult and child part of the personality through drama, dancing, painting or writing.

Writing or journal keeping can give your inner child a voice. My own inner child rebelled, grabbed me by the throat and poured out a stream of complaints in writing about two years ago. It came in what seemed like poetry and this mystified me because I knew nothing about writing in this form and have never taken any interest in poetry. In fact, until eight years ago the only writing I had done of any kind since nursing days was a shopping list or an entreaty to some teacher to save one of my offspring from some hated physical activity!

My inner child must have been an opportunist; since I always have a pencil in my hand she became my Muse. My weariness on my own inward journey promoted this.

## Wouldn't It Be Easy

If we could just call Mr Dyno-rod
When expression freezes
And moribund feelings choke our life canal;
A banal thought, perhaps,

But if he could poke and prod
And suddenly, if without fears or tears,
All that greasy-grime of gruelling years
Could go with a glorious glug down the plug,
Wouldn't it be nice.

It would also be nice
Not to have to pay the price

To be a pilgrim.

I believe that through the inner child we have access not only to whom we really are but also that this is our direct communication with our God-spark, our soul, spirit, psyche, and if we have not integrated this with our personality how can we reach further and connect with our Creator, God, Allah, The Great White Spirit, Universal Energy, Unconditional Love – the Love that passes all understanding, or whatever name you give the Divine? If you are cut off from yourself, how can you love God, how can you love your fellow human beings? Jung calls the process of bringing the soul and the personality together 'individuation'. It can be a battle.

How can I nurture this child
Sickly, yet wild with a strength
Which has me beaten; I know she's just.

But I'm weary of her uprightness, her persistence.

## *Be yourself not what others think you should be*

Laughter is a great defence against panic. It provides an internal massage and releases tension. Here is a little story I have written about Terence, who loved himself just as he was. I hope it might make you smile.

### *Terence the Tiger*

I'm Terence the tiger,
A tiger gone wrong.
I'm not bold, I'm not fierce, I'm not snarling.

111

I'm kind and polite, a furry delight,
And always everyone's darling.
I love bunny rabbits, and chipmunks and frogs,
And cute little kittens, and bold little dogs.
Folks can laugh, they can jeer, they can tease or deride,
*I am what I am,* marshmallow inside.
They can point, they can wink, or shout namby pamby,
I refuse to eat deer; could you eat a Bambi?

I'll feed on mashed swede and the love that abounds
And have Tigger to tea when my birthday comes round.


May the love and light
of the Creator shine
on you as your journey
towards self and The Infinite.


Poems from an unpublished collection *Finding the Thou in You.*

# Further Reading

Budd, Martin L., *Low Blood Sugar: How to understand and overcome hypoglycaemia*. Thorsons, London, new edn 1998.

Chopich, Erika J., and Paul, Margaret, *Healing Your Aloneness: Finding love and wholeness through your inner child*. Harper & Row, New York, 1990.

Conley, Rosemary, *New Inch Loss Plan*. Arrow, London, second revised edn 1998.

Davies, Stephen, and Stewart, Alan, *Nutritional Medicine*. Pan Books, London, 1987.

Downing, Damien, *Daylight Robbery: The importance of sunshine to health*. Arrow, London, revd edn 1998.

Hawkins, Margaret, *Overcoming Panic and Related Anxiety Disorders*. Sheldon Press, London, 2008.

Hay, Louise, *You Can Heal Your Life*. Eden Grove Editions, Enfield, 1984, revd edn 1988.

Janov, Arthur, *The Primal Scream: primal therapy, the cure for neurosis*. Kessinger Publishing, Whitefish, 2007.

Jeffers, Susan, *Feel the Fear and Do It Anyway*. Arrow, 1987, special 20th anniversary edn Vermilion, 2007.

Krieger, Dolores, *The Therapeutic Touch: How to use your hands to help or to heal*. Prentice Hall, New Jersey, 1979.

Kushi, Michio, and John David Mann, *Diabetes and Hypoglycaemia: A natural approach*. Japan Publications Trading Co., Tokyo, 1985.

Lader, Professor Malcolm, *Tranquillizers and Antidepressants: When to take them, how to stop*. Sheldon Press, London, 2008.

Lowen, Alexander, *Bioenergetics*. Penguin, New York, 1979.

Murphy, Melissa, *Overcoming Agoraphobia*. Sheldon Press, London, 2008.

Neville, Alice, *Who's Afraid? Coping with fear, anxiety and panic attacks*. Arrow, London, 1991.

Peck, Scott M., *The Road Less Travelled*. Arrow, London, 1978, special 25th anniversary edn Rider, 2003.

Searle, Ruth, *Overcoming Shyness and Social Anxiety*. Sheldon Press, London, 2008.

Shone, Neville, *Chronic Pain Diet Book*. Sheldon Press, London, 2008.

Soyka, Fred, *The Ion Effect: How air electricity rules your life and health*. London, Bantam, 1978, revd edn 1991.

Tisserand, Maggie, *Aromatherapy for Women*. Thorsons, London, 1985, revd edn Healing Arts Press, Vermont, 1996.

Trickett, Shirley, *Coping with Anxiety and Depression*. Sheldon Press, London, 1989.

Trickett, Shirley, *Irritable Bowel Syndrome and Diverticulosis*. Thorsons, London, 1990, revd edn 1999.

Weekes, Claire, *Self Help for Your Nerves*. London, Collins Fontana, 1992.

Yudkin, John, *Pure, White and Deadly: The problem of sugar*. Viking, London, 1988.

# Useful Addresses

**Association for Neuro-Linguistic Programming (ANLP)**
41 Marlowes
Hemel Hempstead
Herts HP1 1LD
Tel.: 0845 053 1162
Website: www.anlp.org

Neuro-Linguistic Programming is a powerful body of information about how the human mind works. At its heart is a wide range of methods and models for understanding how people think, behave and change. NLP practitioners offer, among other things, a form of counselling which often produces relief from post-traumatic stress, phobias and other anxiety problems. The Association also publishes *Rapport*, a quarterly magazine which is free to members or available by subscription.

**Battle Healthy Living Clinic**
Penny Davenport
Woodlands
London Road
Battle
East Sussex TN33 0LP
Tel.: 01424 773373
Website: www.battlehealthylivingclinic.co.uk

For advice by experienced nutritionists on all aspects of nutrition including special diets, colon cleansing, natural health and skin care.

**BioCare Ltd**
Lakeside
180 Lifford Lane
Kings Norton

Birmingham B30 3NU
Tel.: 0121 433 3727
Website: www.biocare.co.uk

Suppliers of a wide range of nutritional supplements.

**City of London Migraine Clinic**
22 Charterhouse Square
London EC1M 6DX
Tel.: 020 7251 3322
Website: www.colmc.org.uk

**The Council for Information on Tranquillisers and Antidepressants (CITA)**
JDI Centre
3–11 Mersey View
Waterloo
Liverpool L22 6QA
Tel.: 0151 474 9626
Helpline: 0151 932 0102 (10 a.m. to 1 p.m., daily)
Website: www.citawithdrawal.org.uk

**First Steps to Freedom**
PO Box 476
Newquay
Cornwall TR7 1WQ
Helpline: 0845 120 2916
Website: www.first-steps.org

A charity helping phobics, anxiety sufferers and their carers.

**Herbs of Grace**
20 Merlin Park
Fred Dennatt Way
Mildenhall
Suffolk IP28 7RD
Tel.: 01638 712123
Website: www.herbsofgrace.co.uk

**Life Tools**
39 Clive Avenue
Baddely Green
Stoke on Trent ST2 7HR
Tel.: 01782 644008
Website: www.lifetools.com

Suppliers of relaxation aids, such as the MindLab, a small compact machine which works with light and sound frequencies, using lightframes and earphones, to alter brainwave patterns to promote relaxation and sleep, or to raise energy or concentration levels. Can be extremely effective for tension.
**Warning: the MindLab is not for use by those with epilepsy.**

**National Phobics Society**
Zion Community Resource Centre
339 Stretford Road
Hulme
Manchester M15 4ZY
Tel.: 0870 7700 456
Website: www.phobics-society.org.uk

**No Panic**
93 Brands Farm Way
Telford
Shropshire TF3 2JQ
Tel.: 01952 590005
Helpline: 0808 808 0545
Website: www.nopanic.org.uk

**Nutrition Associates Ltd**
Galtres House
Lysander Close
York YO30 4XB
Tel.: 01904 691591
Website: www.naltd.co.uk

Offers medical advice and treatment based on nutrition and allergy principles.

**Relaxation for Living Institute**
1 Great Chapel Street
London W1F 8FA
Tel.: 020 7439 4277
Website: www.rfli.co.uk

This charity helps people to be less anxious and tense. There is an online shop with details of books, audio products and DVDs, and they run small-group classes around the UK.

**Weight Watchers**
Millennium House
Ludlow Road
Maidenhead
Berkshire SL6 2SL
Tel.: 07900 494 736
Website: www.weightwatchers.co.uk

# Index

ear, inner 13
electrical field 107
emotional health 23–4, 81
energy 66
Euhypnos (temazepam) 42, 54
exercise 15, 101–3
exercises: agoraphobia 94;
    blood circulation 102;
    breathing 69–73; electrical
    field 106–7; stretching 66;
    tension releasing 80–9;
    therapeutic touch 107–8

fainting 11, 24
fasting 13
fats 46, 75
fear 9–10, 79
fluorescent lights 62
Frisium (clobazam) 54

glands: adrenal 46, 50;
    pituitary 50
glucose 41, 46
glucose tolerance 43
Glucose Tolerance Factor 77
Glucose Tolerance Test 44–5
glycogen 46
GP 16–17, 91
grounding 82

hallucinations 33
hangover 49
headaches 22, 60–1
    see also migraine
heat 15
heroin 44
histamine 104
homoeopathy 60
hyperactivity 24

hyperglycaemia 47
hypoglycaemia 41–2, 47–8

insomnia 23
insulin 41, 47–8
ionizers 61–2, 105
ions 61–2, 104–6
irritability 23
Irritable Bowel Syndrome 105

jet lag 15, 61–2

Krieger, Dolores 106

laughter 89, 111–12
libido 23
Librium (chlordiazepoxide) 54
liver 46
Lum, Professor L. C. 30, 39
lungs 67–8
lymphatic system 22, 79, 101

magnesium 59, 77
massage 85–8, 101, 106
ME 101
migraine 49
Mogadon (nitrazepam) 42, 54
muscles 22–3, 28, 79–90

nerves 15, 21–4
nervous breakdown 80
nicotine 57–9
Normison (temazepam) 42, 54
nose, stuffy 15
nurse-therapist 18

oil: evening primrose 77; olive
    75